Autobiography
of a Persistent
Anesthesiologist

Autobiography
of a Persistent
Anesthesiologist

Edmond I "Ted" Eger, II, MD

EDITORS

Steven L. Shafer, MD

Lynn Spitler, MD

Wolters Kluwer

Philadelphia · Baltimore · New York · London
Buenos Aires · Hong Kong · Sydney · Tokyo

Acquisitions Editor: Keith Donnellan
Senior Development Editor: Ashley Fischer
Marketing Manager: Kirstin Wartud
Production Project Manager: Justin Wright
Design Coordinator: Stephen Druding
Manufacturing Coordinator: Beth Welsh
Prepress Vendor: TNQ Technologies

9 8 7 6 5 4 3 2 1

Printed in China

Library of Congress Cataloging-in-Publication Data

ISBN-13: 978-1-975169-19-0

Cataloging in Publication data available on request from publisher.

shop.lww.com

CCS0721

To Lynn
and my children

Table of Contents

My darling husband, Ted, started writing his autobiography after his book *The Wondrous History of Anesthesia* was published in 2014.[1] Ted and his coeditors, Larry Saidman and Rod Westhorpe, worked on Wondrous for 6 years. Writing this foreword, I discovered anew Ted's inscription on the first page of Wondrous:

> To Lynn –
> *Oh, wondrous wife of mine*
> *Who gave me gifts of infinite time,*
> *And support during my losses and gains,*
> *And griefs and gambles and growing pains,*
> *Telling a life loved and lived anew;*
> *This is a book I've shared with you.*
> *Much love,*
> *Ted*

This is equally true of his autobiography. In these pages, Ted tells of a life loved and lived anew. As I edit the text in the early morning hours, I hear his voice next to me, joyfully sharing this story of his life.

Ted's family and close friends might be perplexed (but not really) as to why he devoted so much of the text to the science of anesthetic pharmacology. Why did he delve into MAC, pharmacokinetics, and mechanisms of anesthetic action in such detail? Conversely, anesthesiologists might wonder why he bothered talking about his mom and dad, instead of focusing on how he came to understand pharmacokinetics. The answer to both questions is the same. This is Ted's story. His science was inseparable from his life.

Ted discusses this in his epilogue, but I think it's important to introduce Ted at the beginning. As Ted notes, his version of "love me, love my dog" would be "love me, love my science." The science of his life was so interwoven with his personal and family life; Ted saw it as all one story.

As Ted's wife, and as an observer of his scientific passion, there is another reason that Ted wove family and science into one story. Ted brought his unique persona, in full force, to everything he did. He was passionately committed to excellence. Many readers will appreciate how his passion for excellence drove his scientific adventures. However, he was equally passionate about his personal life. He held his role as a father and husband every bit as dear as his role as a clinician, a teacher, and a scientist. Every aspect of his life received the full "Ted Eger" treatment. That is why this is one story.

Ted's autobiography explains his lifetime commitment to training anesthesia researchers. In these pages, Ted illustrates the struggles and rewards that await young investigators. In high school, Ted was an inferior student. He struggled mightily to improve his academic record. As Ted notes in his epilogue, he transformed his life through a combination of persistence and ambition. Ted readily acknowledged that he also benefited from good luck: training at the University of Iowa, meeting John Severinghaus, settling at UCSF. Together, these create a template for young anesthesiologists. You will need persistence, a great mentor, a conducive environment, luck, and ambition.

Ted and I enjoyed 21 wonderful years together. I'm grateful for that. His autobiography also speaks to my own hopes. I hope someone can develop a better early diagnostic test for pancreatic cancer. I'm grateful for my 21 years with Ted, but I would have joyfully welcomed 21 more.

Lynn Spitler, MD

Reference

1. Eger EI, Saidman LJ, Westhorpe R. The wondrous story of anesthesia New York: Springer, 2014.

Ted died on August 26, 2017 of pancreatic cancer, at the age of 86. In his passing, as in his life, Ted got the last word. Ted regularly composed poetry. The day after he passed, a poem mysteriously arrived at his home:

TO LYNN

The time has arrived
My darling wife
For me to depart
This wondrous life.

Please have no fears
Please shed no tears
Hold tight to the memories
Of our 21 years.

Of work and travels
Of books and discoveries
Of hiking and cribbage
Of loving and poetries.

But life is for living
And on you must go
Continue with passion
Til the end of the show.

Throw open the windows
Feel the breeze, wild and free
I'll be soaring above
Loving you abundantly.

When your sand runs low
And others have wept
My embrace welcomes you
Our promises kept.

—Ted 2017

Most knew Ted as a revered scientist and respected colleague. Few knew the sweet, kind, gentle, and profoundly sentimental husband and father. To understand this side of Ted, turn ahead to page 133. The poem he wrote to Lynn on his marriage is "Promises."

On February 2, 2018, UCSF held the Ted Eger Memorial Symposium to celebrate his life and contributions to pharmacology, anesthesiology, and the delivery of safe anesthesia to every patient requiring surgery. Friends and colleagues travelled from all over the world to celebrate his life.

Ted was a founder and lifelong supporter of WARC, the Western Anesthesia Resident's Conference. Recognizing his dedication to resident teaching, WARC established a lectureship in his name. The Northwestern University Feinberg School of Medicine, from which he graduated, will name a professorship in his honor (they are looking for an appropriately distinguished candidate as this goes to press).

Ted's first great-grandchild was born in 2018.

With the urging of Ted's wife, Lynn Spitler, and his dear friend and colleague, Larry Saidman, a reluctant Ted Eger began working on his autobiography in 2015. About a year later Ted asked if I would serve as his editor. Ted is one of my mentors, role models, and heroes. Honored to be asked, I gladly accepted.

Over the next 10 months Ted sent me rough chapters sprinkled with pictures. I edited and revised his text with caution and a little apprehension. Ted was a precise and accurate writer. He was also the world's expert on anesthetic uptake and distribution. I rearranged much of the text, wove the pictures into the manuscript, and added some color of my own (which he accepted with amusement). Every chapter went back and forth between us until Ted was happy with the final product.

Readers will notice that the narrative veers toward a textbook style review when Ted discusses his fundamental contributions to anesthetic pharmacology. Ted didn't cut and paste these from a textbook. Ted wrote these chapters *de novo* to share his life's story. In these chapters, you hear Ted's voice, echoing lectures he gave hundreds of times. The science of anesthetic pharmacology was so woven into the fabric of Ted's life that the two are inseparable, even in the autobiography.

On Saturday, July 15, 2017 Ted and I spent 6 hours working on Chapter 8, The Evolution of Pharmacokinetics. This was the most difficult chapter. With considerable back-and-forth, we turned a comprehensive scientific review into a more personal narrative.

The following day we saw Hamilton (**Figure 1**). Ted wasn't feeling particularly well. Pamela (my wife and another of Ted's mentees) had to tickle him to elicit his usual grin. The play was particularly poignant, ending with "Who lives, who dies, who tells your story?"

Ted tells his story in the pages of this autobiography. On August 7, Ted sent me his approval of the final edits of the epilogue. Ted passed away, at his home, on August 26. His family was with him. The first use of Ted's autobiography was to prepare material for his obituaries.[1,2]

Ted wisely recruited Lynn Spitler and Larry Saidman as reviewers. Both spent many hours reviewing the chapters before sending them to me. I recruited my wife, Pamela Flood, to provide an additional review of the chapters. Tom Hornbein filled in details about the ascent of Mount Rainier, and helped proofread the final text. Ted's children and their spouses spent many hours reviewing the text and offering suggestions.

The final work represents the sustained commitment of Lynn, who meticulously reviewed every word on Ted's behalf.

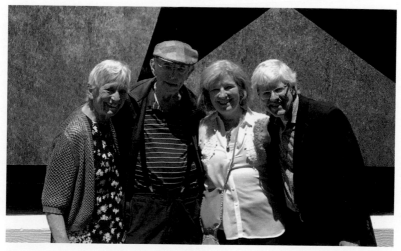

Figure 1   Lynn, Ted, and Pamela Flood at Hamilton, June 16, 2017.

Ted contributed to the lives of everyone he touched. He improved the safety of anesthesia for every person on the planet. His contributions to anesthesia will last to the end of human existence.

He will always be one of my dearest friends.

Steven L. Shafer, MD

References

1. https://www.nytimes.com/2017/09/20/obituaries/dr-edmond-eger-ii-86-dies-found-way-to-make-anesthesia-safer.html
2. Gropper MA, Shafer SL. Dr Ted Eger Obituary. *Anesth Analg*. 2017;125:1829-1830.

At the request of Drs Eger, Shafer, and Spitler, all royalties from Autobiography of a Persistent Anesthesiologist are paid to the Foundation for Anesthesia Education and Research (FAER).

Birth and Early Education

> *I was born about ten thousand years ago,*
> *And there's nothin' in this world I don't know.*
> *I saw Peter, Paul and Moses*
> *Play'n ring around the roses,*
> *And I'll whup the guy that says it isn't so.*
>
> —*Carl Sandburg*

I was born on Wednesday, September 3, 1930, in Michael Reese Hospital, Chicago, 84 years after Morton's 1846 discovery and demonstration of the anesthetic effects of diethyl ether. I arrived in life midway between today and that momentous discovery, a discovery that underlies my self-identity. At the time of my birth, anesthesia as a medical discipline had lived half its life, having changed modestly, or not at all, from the days of Wells, Morton, and Snow. Nitrous oxide and "*ether*" (diethyl ether) continued as the primary general anesthetics. Anesthesia adjustments were based on the patient's response as described in Snow's "*degrees of anesthesia*" or Guedel's later "*signs and stages of anesthesia.*" Waters had just established the world's first Department of Anesthesiology at the University of Wisconsin. Most patients breathed spontaneously during anesthesia rather than being ventilated. Tracheal tubes were used rarely. The half-century that followed completed the transformation of anesthesia from an art into a discipline based on science.

My Family and Early Schooling

My family structure tracked the social norms of the day. My father, Edmond, was the family breadwinner (**Figure 1.1**). He founded an advertising agency, C & E (Crittenden and Eger), which he eventually ran as chief executive and sole director.

Earlier in life he dreamt of being a physician. He enrolled in medical school at the University of Chicago, but withdrew after one semester because of a peculiar neurosis: he feared fainting when asked a question in class.

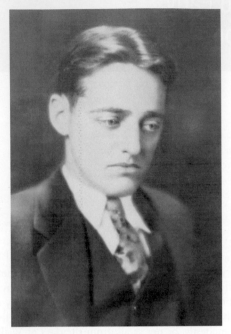

Figure 1.1   My father, perhaps shortly after he left medical school.

My mother, Miriam (**Figures 1.2** and **1.3**), managed our household affairs. She ran our house well. I believe she loved me and wanted to be a source of warmth and support. However, for unclear reasons, I didn't embrace the love and affection she offered. I felt closer to my father (**Figure 1.4**).

Our family lived in an apartment building in Chicago on Ingleside Avenue, a building owned by my grandfather, Emil (**Figure 1.5**). Emil and his wife, my grandmother Sophie, lived in a nearby apartment in the same building. Our family was assisted by a live-in cook. While my parents weren't wealthy, they had enough money to hire help at Depression-era wages.

My mother coordinated visits to our elderly relatives who lived in the same apartment building owned by my grandfather, or in maroon velvet-walled rooms in upscale residential hotels in affluent areas of Chicago. She also arranged holidays, picnics, and trips to the zoo. She even sent me to camp, which, a sissy at the mercy of bullies, I detested. I still hate them.

I knew no specifics of what my mother did during the day other than running the house. She pursued activities related to her interests in piano, singing, and

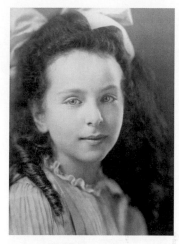

Figure 1.2   My mother as a girl.

acting. Prior to her marriage, her acting interest had led to a trip to Hollywood. She was offered an introductory role in exchange for a suitable *"casting couch"* finder's fee. She declined the offer, returned to Chicago, accepted my father's proposal of marriage, and assumed her role as wife and then mother. She was involved in a few local opera productions, none of which I saw.

As a young child, I was closest to my grandfather, Emil (**Figure 1.6**). At the time (1930-1935), four Eger families (**Figure 1.7**) lived in his apartment

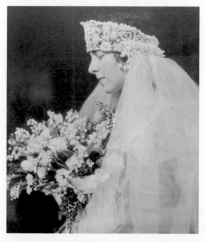

Figure 1.3   My mother as a bride.

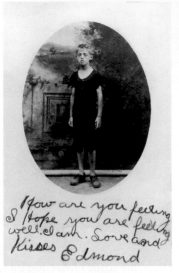

*How are you feeling
I Hope you are feeling
well. I am. Love and
Kisses   Edmond*

Figure 1.4   A postcard from my father.

complex: my family, his family, and uncles Albert Eger and Alex Eger. Emil and his brothers Albert and Alex were born in the prior century in Presov, Hungary.

Each evening, Emil would come home and listen to the news on the radio. When the news was over, Grandfather Emil and I would play a game of casino for vast sums of money. I was a great casino player. I never lost, collecting penny after penny. *Where did he get all those pennies?* My grandfather was generous with his pennies, but even more so with his time. As a child with preoccupied parents, having grandpa play casino each evening made me feel valued. He manipulated each game in my favor. *Sly fox!* Looking back, I appreciate his wile.

Emil took me for walks and for summer forays on Chicago's open-air double-decker buses. Sometimes, for fun, he would draw pictures, maps of an imagined boy's journey, complete with falling into holes and climbing mountains. As he drew, the path taken by the boy became the outline of an animal. Emil lifted me up, made me important, and changed my life. He taught me that winning was fun, and that I could do it!

Emil had two children by his first wife, Hermia: Edmond (my father) and Ruth (my aunt). Hermia died before I was born. I knew Emil's second wife, Sophia Wieger, who passed away when I was 13 years old.

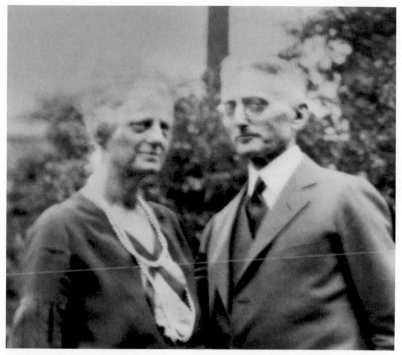

Figure 1.5   Emil Eger with his wife Sophie.

Emil owned three cigar stores and sold tobacco until late in life, when he was driven out of business by the arrival of cigar store chains. Tobacco led to more than business disappointment. His smoking produced increasingly severe coronary artery disease. Emil turned to my father, with his one semester of medical education, for his recommendations on how Emil might relieve the pain in his chest.

Emil was the magician of my life. One day, when I was 15 years old, the magician disappeared. I didn't know how much I had lost with his death.

I was not as close to my maternal grandparents, Edward and Bertha Newmann (**Figure 1.8**). Edward demanded displays of affection, which I provided grudgingly and secretly resented. Edward's father, Bernhard Newmann, my maternal great-grandfather, was a saloon keeper. Edward didn't follow his father in the saloon business, becoming a successful lawyer instead. Edward and Bertha had three daughters: Miriam (my mother), her older sister Jewel Carolyn (a renegade Bohemian, who changed her name to Michael J. Adams following a divorce), and Betty (the sweetest of the lot).

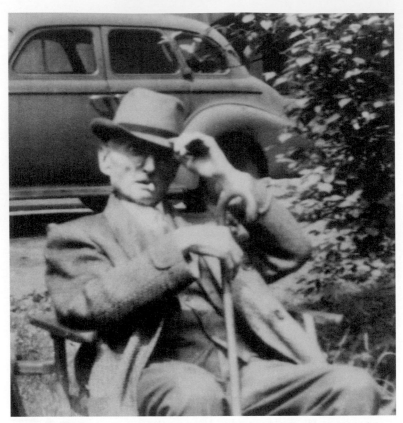

Figure 1.6 Emil with cigarette. I know he smoked and owned cigar stores, but I don't remember that he smoked when he was with me.

Edward played pinochle with cronies in smoky rooms. But Edward the rogue (I call him now) had redeeming graces. He wrote poems, including a long one for children about a magical land. For all I knew he never wrote another poem, but the existence of even one epic poem suggests I probably misjudged him.

Aunt Betty met and married Harry Geiger (**Figure 1.9**). They didn't live happily forevermore, but for a time they were more than content to share a life. I was pleased to share some of it with them.

My parents married in 1929, and I was born in 1930. My sister Conni was born in 1935, when I was 5 years old. I think Conni's arrival prompted my parents' decision to move in the late 1930s. I recall overhearing my mother

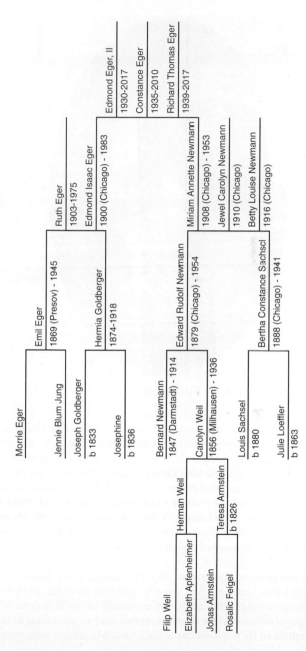

Figure 1.7 Eger family tree.

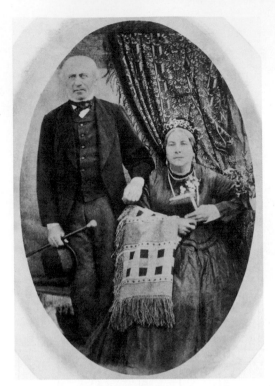

Figure 1.8   Grandpa Edward Newmann and his wife Bertha.

negotiating with the owner for the purchase of the house that would become our new home, a three-story beauty on Ellis Avenue (**Figure 1.10**). The first floor of our new house comprised the living-music room, dining room, break-fast room, pantry, and kitchen. Our family occupied bedrooms on the second floor, where my father's study-office was also located. The staff lived on the third floor. My mother directed the work of a housekeeper, a cook, and a nanny who looked after Conni and me. Housework was delegated to the staff. My mother cared for the phlox garden. She enjoyed gardening, but not weeding. She paid me a penny for every 10 weeds I pulled to help her.

My parents also paid me a penny for each fly I caught in the house. Budding capitalist that I was, I used my first wages to purchase fly-paper, vastly increas-ing my earnings. I caught flies in the house, mostly in the basement. When I and my fly-paper exhausted that supply, I opened the basement door to the out-side and diminished fly numbers in the back yard. My parents soon discovered

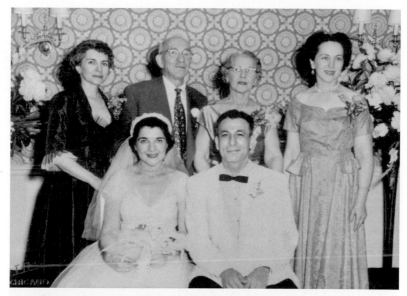

Figure 1.9   Harry Geiger marries aunt Betty (front row). The back row from left to right are aunt Michael, grandpa Edward Newmann, his new wife Kitty Ziv, and my mother, Miriam.

my subterfuge. They were impressed with my ingenuity rather than angered by my deceit, but the monetary return on flies disappeared.

My brother, Tom, was born in 1939. Since our house had four bedrooms, a study, and a sleeping porch on the second floor, Tom had his own bedroom from infancy. The age separation with Tom precluded our becoming close as children, just as it had with Conni. With a large house, and chores mostly designated to the household staff, we lived together as a family without establishing close bonds of mutual support.

School

My parents could afford sending me to the Hyde Park School for Little Children at the age of 3. I remember developing an intimate relationship with Dick and Jane, dazzled by the connection between the language I spoke and the written word. It pleased me to find that collections of letters had meaning. In addition to the library's children's books, my classroom held a child-sized cardboard house with chairs for 3- or 4-year-old students. This little house was the prize for the child who finished his lessons first. It was invariably mine to claim, perhaps the longest winning streak of my life!

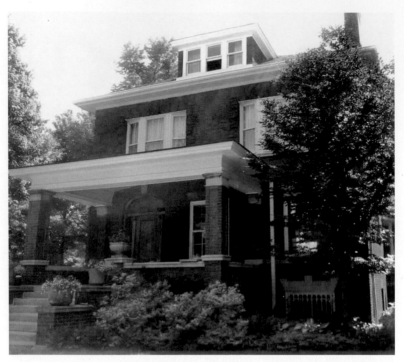

Figure 1.10   The house at 5039 Ellis Avenue in Chicago. To the left and unseen was a brick fence that separated our house from the Loeb house, of Leopold and Loeb fame.

I often visited grandmother Sophie in her nearby apartment. Sophie, a retired schoolteacher, supplemented my arithmetic lessons. She taught me multiplication tables and the magic of the factor of 10. To a young child 12 × 12 seemed hard. Sophie taught me to reduce a single hard problem to two easy problems: 12 × 10 plus 12 × 2. 120 + 24 = 144. *Oh, how easy! Why isn't arithmetic taught this way?*

I entered Charles Kozminski public elementary school as a stellar student. My preparation at Hyde Park School for Little Children was good enough for me to skip kindergarten. I could probably have skipped more than that, as I was reading at a seventh-grade level. However, for reasons not clear to me even now, I rapidly sank to the bottom of my class. Perhaps it was because I was about a-year-and-a-half younger than my classmates. Regardless of the reason, I remained stuck in academic doldrums for a decade. I failed courses repeatedly. I could not describe the structure of a sentence. I failed to understand fractions. I did not comprehend science. I failed nearly everything except Mrs. Ray's class in art. *Dear Mrs. Ray, did I ever adequately thank you?* Despite terrible academic performance, my teachers dutifully passed me from grade to grade.

The issue was not that I rebelled against learning. Quite the contrary—I read and read. I read books on mythology, fairy tales, stories of animals (*Lassie Come Home; Call of the Wild*). One of my present treasures is a copy of *English Fairy Tales*, a book of bloody stories that I stole from our school library, a book whose cover disintegrated and, years later, was lovingly replaced by my eldest daughter, Cris. I lost myself in these images where boys and men were masters and adventurers. I loved comic books, learning the word "bizarre" from Superman.

I discovered the world of science. Books on chemistry and physics and medical heroes appeared on my bookshelf adjacent to Superman and Lassie. I devoured books by Paul de Kruif about scientist-physicians who conquered disease and famine, particularly *Microbe Hunters, Hunger Fighters,* and *Men Against Death*. I had dreams of becoming one of them, a Robert Koch or Ignaz Semmelweis, performing simple experiments with results that saved thousands of lives. De Kruif made it sound so easy. Even a country physician like Koch could become a great scientist. (And, of course, my father would have been pleased to have me become a physician!)

My buddies and I would scramble over fences and across yards, exploring. My mother rescued me from my misadventures. On one occasion, we climbed atop a peaked commercial greenhouse. The owner appeared, shaking his fist at us, demanding that we get down. And so, we did. I slid down one side while my buddies slid down the other, breaking windows as we went. The buddies escaped, but I was caught. The furious owner direly predicted my behavior would land me in reform school. It sounded terrible. Mother appeared (**Figure 1.11**) and soon we left. *Thank God, no reform school!* We got into the car. Head down, I awaited being chastised. Instead, having gotten safely away from the greenhouse owner and reform school, my mother collapsed in laughter.

I was not surprised by my mother's reaction. Growing up, I was disciplined minimally or not at all. My parents generally encouraged good acts by approval and reason. However, between roughly my fifth and tenth years, they began adding corporal punishment for egregious acts such as putting water into the wooden sandbox (bad because the sandbox would rot). My mother would ask my father to apply corporal punishment when she deemed some infraction appropriately heinous ("*a spanking when your father gets home*"). Truly dangerous acts (eg, my accidentally setting the kitchen curtains afire) went unpunished. The only other punishment I remember occurred on a Christmas when I received coal and lemons rather than presents. They withdrew the punishment when I repented whatever egregious act had led to the coal and lemons.

My mother defended me, her genius son, for my failures at school. I overheard her argue with a teacher that I couldn't possibly be incompetent in fractions. She was wrong. I was an exemplar for incompetency. However, she made little effort to understand, or correct, what had gone wrong after my graduation

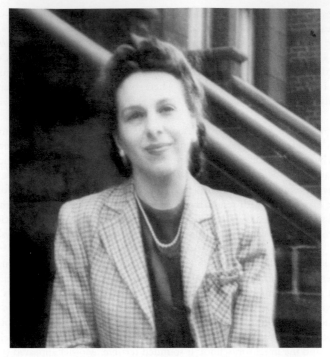

Figure 1.11   My mother, Miriam, at roughly the time I slid down the greenhouse roof.

from the Hyde Park School for Little Children. She did get a tutor who taught me Spanish and helped me pass the next year of that subject…but just barely. I abandoned Spanish and took up French and got equally poor grades. *Good Lord, why did I think French would be easier than Spanish?*

I ended my first semester in junior high school with three D's (for science, algebra, and English) and an F (Spanish). The D's probably were gifts. I seemed not to have the capacity for memorization that each class required. Despite the D in science, I liked the chemistry books I read. I also liked making explosives. I learned how to mix nitrates and sulfur to wondrous effect, pursuing experiments that might have destroyed our house.

I didn't get low grades in every class. Ms. Minnie Moore, a diminutive teacher and famous for odd things made geometry a revelation. Against the rules, the boys might toss a football in the hall. Coming from nowhere and jumping far beyond her 5-foot height, Ms. Moore would intercept the pass and disappear with the ball. Until the second year of high school, I had assumed that all problems could be reasoned to a solution, not understanding that sometimes memorization was required (explaining my failure to pass Spanish and other courses). For reasons now lost, I memorized the basic theorems of geometry, the limited number of fundamental principles from which the entire subject derived. Perhaps I remembered them because the principles were so few. Perhaps I remembered them because I intuited that they were fundamentally true and was drawn to the rightness of those principles. I then discovered, to my amazement, that everything in geometry could be deduced from these principles. Reason could guide me to a correct solution. *A joy!* Ms. Moore gave me a rare "A" grade. I don't know if the pleasure arose from her gift or geometry's elegance, but I suspect the latter.

This pleasure in learning can go too far. By the time I reached college, I had come to love mathematics, getting A's in every course I enrolled in. I took a course in algebra, just for fun, acing each examination, anticipating an easy A. *But no, a B!* "*Why?*" I asked the teacher, who had made mathematics her life. "*Because,*" she replied, "*you didn't take it seriously!*" She was correct; I took it for fun. But I'm getting ahead of the story.

I remember going weekly to the Frolic Theater with my friends and a dime. But one day, the Frolic raised admission from 10c to 11c, and I didn't have the extra penny.

In high school, I noticed an increasing interest in girls. Millions of years of evolution, genetic programming, and rising hormones pushed me in ways I did not understand and could not control. I remember taking my first date to the Frolic Theater. I thought I was expected to hold hands with the girl. *How? Tightly or loosely?* My palms were wet from anxious sweat. *Was that okay? What was the purpose of this hand holding? Was she expecting me to grab her hand, or should I ask permission? Why wasn't this explained in the books on my shelf?* My sexual education proceeded in fits and starts. I received no guidance or instruction from anyone. I managed the testosterone rages that distracted my thoughts and clouded my judgment as well as I could, just as most boys do.

My Father and Checkers

Growing up, I saw little of my father. He enjoyed his work and took his responsibilities as the breadwinner seriously. He worked outside the home, while my mother and her staff raised the children. As the breadwinner, he supplied all my material needs. As noted above, although raised in the heart of the Great Depression, our household staff included a nanny (we called her a nurse), a housekeeper, and a cook. Labor was cheap.

On a few occasions, I visited my father's office at the C & E advertising agency. I was given the job of office boy, tasked with triaging and discarding old files. These included advertisements written by my father promoting Redman Tobacco, embalming fluids, and floor waxes.

My father's biggest account was Admiral Radio and Television. We owned Admiral radios, and later an Admiral television set. The television was in the study on the second floor, adjacent to my bedroom. My father enjoyed watching television when he came home from work, but little on television interested his children.

My father occasionally shared his avocations. He loved golf (**Figure 1.12**) and hoped I might join him. His closest friends and business associates were golfing buddies. However, I was an inept player with little desire to learn.

My father bought me toy sailboats, which we took to a pond constructed for such playthings at the foot of the Chicago Beach Hotel. We set the sails and the direction of the rudder and pushed our ship out on the water, hoping for enough wind to carry our vessel to the other side, perhaps 70 ft away. It always did. And sometimes my father would buy a kite, and we would fly it high into the Chicago sky.

Other than these sporadic activities and an occasional visit to a baseball or football game, our relationship primarily consisted of dinner together. My father was seated at the head of the table with my mother to his right. My three siblings and I sat in the remaining chairs. Discussions between my mother and father occupied most of the conversation.

Once dinner was finished, my father quickly retired to his study where he often worked for hours, writing on lined paper supported by a large, yellow and brown, rigid plastic checkerboard held in his lap. One evening, he invited me to play a game of checkers (draughts). I accepted enthusiastically. I was eager

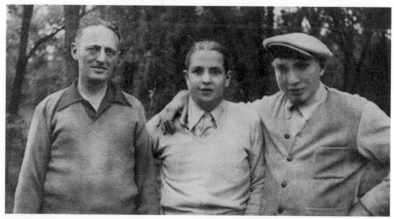

Figure 1.12   Dad (left) with golfing buddies Howard Stern (middle) and best friend Stanton Rose (right).

for his approval and companionship. We played. Unlike his father, Emil, who always steered me to winning, my father had no such intentions. He beat me quickly and easily. However, he did not realize he had opened a magical door. Each evening thereafter, I challenged him to another game. And another. And another. I took playing seriously, even reading the only book I could find on checkers. I still have it: *Tommie Wiswell's Checker Magic.* And shortly, I began to win. I did not expect any gifts from my father, and none were offered. However, we continued playing. Eventually I became unbeatable, winning game after game. A revelation! I had found something I could do well! I insisted on more games, forcing my father's repeated recognition that I was the superior player. I would not lose a game. Not one. I had my second winning streak!

At the age of 13 years, I entered Hyde Park High School, discovering that chess and checkers were among the sports offered. *Sports!* I, this timid weakling, could win an athletic letter! My algebra teacher, Mr. Olmsted (yes, the same Mr. Olmsted!) mentored the chess and checker club. I joined the checker enthusiasts, a distinct minority of the club members. Quickly I established myself as the best checker player in the club. I became the captain of the vaunted Hyde Park High School Checker Team. Although my grades were dismal (I graduated in the bottom 20% of my high school class), I led the team that won the All Chicago Checker Championship 2 years running. Thereafter, two plaques commemorating our triumphs lined the school wall. They may be there today. And I did receive an athletic (!) letter for this success, adding to my sense that I could at least do one thing well.

My father's expectations and my desires ultimately affected both our relationship and how I fared at school. I wanted my father's love and approval. This approval certainly did not come from my grades in elementary school or high school. He made an occasional attempt to guide me, once spending an hour struggling with my inability to solve an algebra problem. Despairing of my ineptitude, he enjoined me to "*THINK!*" I remember him shouting the word, but probably he did not. I hadn't thought to ask him how to think, although it strikes me now as an excellent question.

World War II

I remember exactly when World War II started. On December 7, 1941, we were living in the house on Ellis Avenue. I heard noise from below. I came down the back stairway, as my buddy ran up the stairs yelling *"They bombed Pearl Harbor!"* I asked, *"Where's Pearl Harbor?"* It dominated the news and changed the lives of everyone I knew. However, since I was only 11 years old, and my father was 41 years, the male Eger's were not inducted into the army. Some of my life continued as though nothing had changed, other than the rationing of food, clothes, and gasoline. As manufacturing was directed to the war effort, new cars became unavailable, and old tires were retreaded. The primary change for our family was driven by the war economy. With the country at war and the government paying for skilled labor, Depression-era wages were no longer competitive. Our cook, the nanny, and the housekeeper left for better paying jobs. We had to do the housework ourselves. I cleaned the house, shoveled coal into the furnace, and took out the clinkers.

World War II brought other changes to the Eger family. The war meant employment opportunities for African-Americans, who now could afford homes in our neighborhood. Additionally, the "*gentlemen's agreements*" that white homeowners would only sell to other white homeowners vanished with the changes in social mores. My parents ultimately joined the "*white flight*" to Flossmoor, a whites-only suburb of Chicago. My parents were not overtly bigoted. However, like many of their generation, they felt that acceptance of integration would stigmatize them among their friends and neighbors. Indeed, after he was fired by Admiral Radio and Television (for insufficient obedience to the owner, Ross Saragusa), my father established a second career as the Executive Director of the Chicago Council on Foreign Relations, a position that prompted liberal inclinations, including social relations with many minorities.

Agnes Comes to Live With Us

One night early in the 1940s, a girl named Agnes unexpectedly arrived at our home. Agnes was a high-school teenager whose father, a physician, was a distant cousin of my father. My father knew of her father's declining health. He had agreed to be Agnes' legal guardian, but not her custodian. A farmer named Erickson agreed to be Agnes's custodian when her father passed away. After her father's death, Agnes moved in with Erickson. For reasons I never learned, after several years on the farm she ran away, electing to live with the Eger family. She changed her name to Suzanne Eger (**Figure 1.13**).

Suzanne was an engaging person. She was lively, animated, and had a great sense of humor. She was also observant and smart, later passing easily through a year or two at the University of Chicago. Within the family, Suzanne and I often worked as a team. For example, we complained once too often about the quality of dinner in the early 1940s—ie, during World War II. After that, we were told to prepare our own meals. We were given our ration cards and a budget. We ate a lot of carrots.

I learned a lot from Suzanne. After hearing of my belief in God, she challenged me to offer proof of God's existence. Failing to find any such evidence, I immediately became an atheist. Suzanne became the older sister I had never had, the family member who could provide the guidance and insights into life that I needed. I became closer to Suzanne than to my parents or other siblings.

Mother Becomes Ill and Dies

After our move to Flossmoor, my father's business continued to flourish until he was fired by the owner of Admiral Radio and Television. My mother was not so fortunate. Shortly before the end of World War II she was diagnosed with follicular lymphoblastoma, the most common of the non-Hodgkin's lymphomas. Her disease was diagnosed from a cervical lymph node biopsy, which left her neck partly numb. An indolent disease, it progressed slowly. For many years she continued to engage in things that interested her, even taking up tap-dancing. She only became profoundly ill in her final year of life, 1953.

Despite the considerable love she showed me, I don't remember a closeness to my mother. This differed from her relationship with brother Tom. Many years later, Tom wrote:

> *I spent a lot of time with Mom and felt close to her. We'd go in the back room (I think it had been your bedroom), listen to soap operas, work on jigsaw puzzles, and share in our enthusiasm for coin collecting (I still have both of our collections). She used to get headaches and I'd massage her forehead while she lay on that chaise-lounge she had in their bedroom. In the spring, she'd take me and Conni out of school and drive out to Idlewild (Country Club) and we'd pick flowers. Next day each of us would take flowers to our teachers. There were other little things she did to show me her love. In the fall of 1952, Mom had been bedridden pretty*

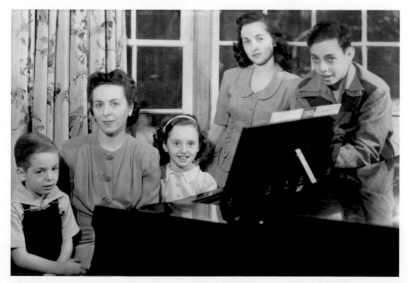

Figure 1.13 From left to right: brother Tom, mother, sister Connie, new sister Suzanne, and me in 1943 in the music room in the house on Ellis Ave.

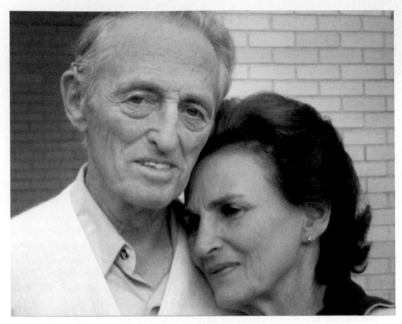

Figure 1.14   My father and Rebecca, his second wife.

much for about 6 months and she just wasn't getting any better. I'd keep innocently suggesting things that might help her get better but somehow I know that either she would get better, or she was going to die, which she did 6 months later. Her last day was dreadful and the memory of it is burned into my mind. No one prepared me for it. I wasn't told until much later that she had lymphoma. They kept those things from you back then.

My mother's death little affected the course of my daily life or that of my siblings. But her death was the source of much grief for my father. In the late 1950s, he married a younger woman, Rebecca (**Figure 1.14**), with whom he fathered my youngest sibling, Larry. I remember being amazed once when my traditional, old-fashioned father referred to his wife, Rebecca, as a *"hot little number."*

Maybe I shouldn't have been surprised. Age is no match for millions of years of evolution and genetic programming.

Epiphany of a Shoe Salesman

I had an epiphany in my junior year in high school. My buddy, Ralph Fertig, suggested that we earn pocket money as Maling's Shoes salesmen. Maling's was one of many low-priced stores on the South Side of Chicago catering to poor, mostly black, women. We applied to Maling's with no experience and were immediately accepted in the labor-short market of the 1940s. My first day I discovered what many shoe salesmen know: women enjoy shoe shopping more than shoe buying. My first day I helped many ladies enjoy the pleasure of trying on pairs of new footwear, but I didn't sell many shoes. My 8 or 10 hours of work left me exhausted. Selling shoes was hard work for little money. I easily connected the trajectory of my academic career with selling shoes…if I didn't improve academically, I might spend my life at Maling's.

That wouldn't do! At this *"ah ha!"* moment, the epiphany of an academic slouch, I resolved to change my trajectory.

Learning to Study

I was poorly positioned to make that change. I had an atrocious academic record. I knew little about the best approaches to study, how to take notes in class, or even what classes to take. I could not get into most institutions of higher learning because of my academic record and the year—1946. Millions of soldiers returning from World War II sought to reestablish their lives by applying for college. Northwestern University, the University of Chicago, and the University of Illinois rejected my applications. The rejection by the University of Chicago galled my father who noted that all the Egers had completed college there with honors. Dad had his Phi Beta Kappa key as proof. And he had been generous in his contributions to the University's endowment. It made no difference; my dismal record spoke too loudly.

A local community college, Roosevelt College (later Roosevelt University) accepted my father's check and me. I enrolled there, highly motivated by carrots (I'd like to be a country physician) and sticks (I did not want to sell shoes). Ralph went as well. I don't know why, because Ralph had the academic qualifications for a better institution. Having never learned how to study, I studied inefficiently. I compensated by studying for longer hours than any sane student would spend. The summer before school I prepared for the classes I would take, reading and rereading the required books. When school began, classes and studying became my life. I slept 4 to 6 hours a night, ate meals, and studied. I studied every day, including holidays. To develop better note-taking skills, I took a course in an off-beat shorthand. It worked, and to this day, I still take notes in shorthand. I was not a brilliant student, but I was a persistent one. Years later I came across a marvelous comment on persistence by an average president, Calvin Coolidge:

> *Nothing in this world can take the place of persistence. Talent will not: nothing is more common than unsuccessful men with talent. Genius will not; unrewarded genius is almost a proverb. Education will not: the world is full of educated derelicts. Persistence and determination alone are omnipotent.*

I had been lucky, by chance hitting on persistence, probably the best approach to study that I could apply. The D's and F's of grammar school and high school became A's in my year at Roosevelt. Armed with A's, the following year I applied and was accepted to the University of Illinois (Chicago and Northwestern still rejected me). The success did wonders for my self-image. Success in school, at Roosevelt, and in my 3 years at the University of Illinois, became an addiction.

A Summer at Columbia University

Academic success was only assured by developing an obsession with course preparation. I studied my courses before taking them. Given my challenges with foreign languages courses, I knew I was in great danger of failing German in my second year of college. In the summer prior to starting at the University of Illinois, I attended summer school at Columbia University to prepare myself to study German. After several weeks, it was clear that I was correct: I indeed had little aptitude for German. I completed the course at Columbia, but took it without credit. That fall I repeated the course at the University of Illinois, scoring an A, the only A I've ever received in a language other than English. I took three more semesters of German. With great effort I managed to get B's.

One of the necessary life skills required to attend Columbia was learning the New York subway system. Exiting one summer evening somewhere near Grand Central Station I found a sign for the New York Chess and Checkers Club. It directed me to the second floor. *Checkers? Yes, checkers!* Played by old men in a smoky room—I stood watching intently, and finally caged a game with one of the old men. I would show him what the captain of the Hyde Park High School

Checker Team could do. But despite great effort, at best I could gain a draw. The old man scarcely looked at the board. This provided a great lesson in humility, and a mini-epiphany. I would not make a living selling shoes or playing checkers.

I'd made friends at Columbia with Kurt Kosterlitz, a classmate and man of the world who took me under his wing. At the summer's end, we drove to Kitty Hawk, North Carolina, staying in a nearly deserted hotel (**Figure 2.1**). Kurt tried to connect me to a thin, red-haired art student. She exuded a scent of sex. I was terrified. Nothing happened despite Kurt's best intentions. I remember drinking beer in a bar at the back of a hotel that bordered the beach with great fondness. I drank to excess and walked out on the beach. The next thing I knew, I was face down in the sand with Kurt kneeling beside me. Later we were warned that a hurricane was coming to Kitty Hawk. As with the red-haired student, nothing came of that either.

An Ascetic Existence

I spent my last 3 years of college at the University of Illinois, where school and grades continued to be the purpose of my life. I was single minded in purpose and continued to be driven by the carrot of a respected career and

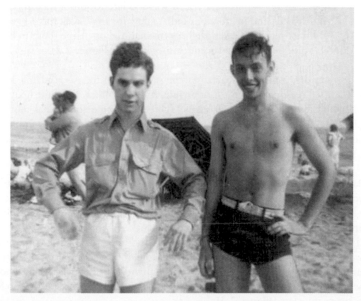

Figure 2.1 Kurt Kosterlitz and me at Kitty Hawk in 1947.

the stick of not wanting to sell shoes. There was no uplifting joy in learning. There was no transcendental beauty in knowledge. It was just school and grades. I chose a major in chemistry and a minor in mathematics. I attended class 12 to 15 hours each day, with an additional 8 to 12 hours of study after class. That adds up to more than 24 hours every day, which is what it usually felt like.

I got a B on my first physics test. Thereafter I slept still less. I would overcome less than perfect grades by working harder, studying longer. Early one morning I found myself holding a ringing alarm clock, trying to connect time, velocity, and acceleration, my mind unable to stop the ringing. But on the next examination, I scored 100, the only student in our class of 600 to do so. Thank God for all those returning veterans. *I called home, triumphant!* My father didn't seem impressed. That came later.

I lived an ascetic existence, a combination of personal choice and the limited accommodations offered by the University of Illinois. Because we had an enormous class, the University could only offer no frills accommodations. Despite our Spartan circumstances, I could tell the University of Illinois was (and continues to be) a superb university.

Since I entered in my sophomore year, I was too late to join a fraternity, and besides, my schedule and inclinations didn't allow for the Greek life. I lived for 2 of my 3 Illinois years in Annex Hall, a gym that had one large room to house 150 double-bunk beds, with adjacent clothes lockers (**Figure 2.2**).

The accommodations were Spartan by the standards of today's academic housing, but it felt reasonable to me for the time. Indeed, it likely felt quite luxurious to the hundreds of returning veterans. There were three communal rooms: a study hall that accommodated half the housed students, bathrooms, and a too-small room for socialization. Our spare accommodations worked well because the mature students it housed made it work well. *They had places to go!*

I clawed at school, this frightening foe that had to be overcome if I were to become a physician. But school had morphed into more than a mere barrier to my becoming a physician. I had to overcome this foe to believe in myself. Bring it on! And I succeeded. I worked around the clock. I went to school year-round and ignored holidays. All seasons. I won A's and an occasional B (*ah, the one in algebra and three later grades in German!*) rolled in. The reward, the sense of triumph, was wonderful. And with awards in hand (Phi Beta Kappa and more, now father was a bit impressed), I graduated at the age of 20 years in the top few percent of my class (**Figure 2.3**).

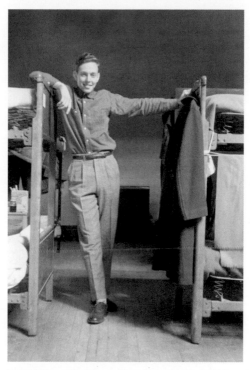

Figure 2.2   I stand between two of the 150 double-bunk beds in Annex Hall.

I applied to medical school at the Northwestern University, the University of Illinois, and the University of Chicago. I was accepted by Northwestern. I never did hear from the University of Illinois. *Perhaps they are still considering my application?* I was rejected outright by the University of Chicago. I didn't take kindly to the rejection (which hasn't changed). Fortunately, revenge came many years later. My brilliant daughter, Renee, applied to the University of Chicago Medical School, was accepted…and chose another medical school. *Ha! Take that, you nasty!*

Ralph and Kurt

Ralph Fertig and I parted company after our year at Roosevelt College. Ralph went to the University of Chicago, where he got a bachelor's degree. He pursued graduate studies in sociology, earning a master's degree from Columbia

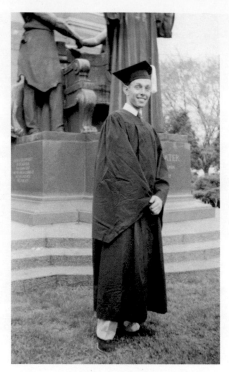

Figure 2.3   At the age of 20 years, I graduated with honors from the University of Illinois.

University and a Doctorate from the University of Chicago. Ralph later called me, now decades ago, from Los Angeles. Other than that one call, we lost track of each other. While writing this part of my autobiography, I wondered if he was still alive. I called Los Angeles information (yes, 411, still works today) and learned that there was only one Ralph Fertig in Los Angeles.

THE Ralph Fertig! We talked for a couple of hours. In high school, I knew Ralph had been a leftward-leaning fellow. I had followed along, joining the ACLU where I did nothing more than pay dues. Still, my ACLU membership got me an interview with the FBI when I was drafted into the US Army. They asked if I was willing to die for my country. I said yes, but I'd prefer not to.

Several months after our recent phone conversation, Ralph and Suzie, his significant other, paid me a visit. We no longer resembled the teenagers who last saw each other. We had lived lives that we shaped, that satisfied us. He was well-regarded as a social justice advocate, speaker, and writer. I learned that he was a more serious liberal than I had previously known. He joined the Freedom Riders in the 1960s. He was jailed in Alabama, where he was beaten, and his ribs fractured. He had gone on to become a lawyer, graduating in the 1970s from UCLA. He became a Professor of Social Studies at the University of Southern California. I admire his courage and bravery, qualities he had in far greater abundance than did I.

Kurt Kosterlitz disappeared from my life after my summer at Columbia University, and magically reappeared as a classmate at Northwestern University Medical School. He was married to a grade schoolteacher. He disappeared again in the middle of his attendance at Northwestern Medical School. I never learned whether he completed medical school. I attempted to track him down and discovered that he had joined the Rotary Club in Morristown, PA. Unfortunately, all they could tell me was that he died there in 1972.

Making Adobes in Baja California

At the University of Illinois, I had attended the Unitarian Church. In my senior year, I applied for one of their summer outreach programs: I would assist building a tuberculosis sanitarium in Mexico. I included this in my application to Northwestern Medical School, not expecting it to be consequential. However, I later learned that Northwestern Medical School had a strong international outreach program for underserved populations. Perhaps my including this tipped the scales for my admission.

Once admitted to medical school, I found myself in the unusual position of not needing to study in the Summer of 1947. Several Unitarian friends and I traveled to Ejido el Porvenir, a small village in Baja, California, near Ensenada. We lived in a local schoolhouse. Together, we fabricated adobes (bricks made from mud, straw, and sun) using large wooden forms that probably had existed for decades. The adobes were large (1 foot by 2 ft by 8 in) and heavy. The houses in Ensenada were all made from such adobes. Each day we made a hundred or more of these. We were guided by the local residents and led by one of the elders, an avuncular man named Gambino.

I missed the opportunity to supplement my limited language skills that summer. I could have and should have learned Spanish. Unfortunately, everyone spoke English. I hadn't the will or foresight to insist upon speaking Spanish. The only expression I learned (or remember) is *"Andalez, andalez, rapido, rapido,"* all with a smile. No one ever translated *"Andalez, andalez, rapido, rapido,"* but surely it means *"Let's go, let's go, quickly, quickly!"*

Seth Arnold was one of my closer friends that summer. We climbed a local mountain and got lost on our return. We carried too little water, and *sin agua* we had put ourselves at risk. As we struggled back, we came upon abandoned farm. We found a well with water, in which a dead rat floated. We made it back without water.

At the end of the summer, the Unitarian Church rewarded us with a tour of Guadalajara and Mexico City. I've not forgotten my introduction to wonderful angry murals by Diego Rivera in Guadalajara. I bought my sophisticated mother a big bright red leather purse. She never used it. In retrospect, I shouldn't be surprised. *A bright red purse? Good grief! What was I thinking?*

Two decades later I returned to Ejido el Porvenir with my family at the time. Gambino was there and so was the building. However, it was no longer a sanitarium. Up to the 1940s, tuberculosis was a terrible scourge, especially for the poor and malnourished. With the development of streptomycin and the 1946 to 1947 proof that it cured tuberculosis—in the first ever randomized double-blind, placebo-controlled study—the need for a sanitarium disappeared. It didn't matter to me. I'd had a wonderful summer making friends. I also cultivated a serious tan that should have been good for several melanomas in later life.

My First Year in Medical School

At the start of my first year of medical school, I joined a fraternity, Phi Rho Sigma. Membership in Phi Rho had several benefits, including social contacts, a library, and the support of those in the fraternity. I had a "big brother," Tom Upton, who was to look out for me, protect me, and guide me. One of his first acts was to steal my girlfriend, Anne, a lovely red-headed freshman, and marry her. They remain married today. He told me that in stealing Anne and marrying her he did me a favor. That's what he told me. I believed him then and still do.

Tom did other good things for me. He recruited me into a barbershop quartet. I could sing well enough, but I read music indifferently. That relegated me to second tenor, the guy who carries the tune because he can't do anything else. Beyond baritone Tom, the other singers were Chuck Lamdin and Ford van Hagen. Chuck was a perfect top tenor. He later became a naval surgeon, probably based on skills other than singing. Ford was the most musically gifted. In addition to singing bass, Ford could write music and lyrics. He composed the lyrics for at least two shows for returning Northwestern alumni, shows in which I sang. In one of these, Ford composed lyrics to be sung to the tune of the quartet from Rigoletto. I gave it my best barbershop voice. My three companions said no, it wouldn't do. It didn't sound like the quartet from any opera. I reached into my memory and belted out my best imitation of a tenor opera singer, dazzling my three friends and me. My performance amazed my mother, who wondered if it really was my voice. To this day I can still sing this odd version of the quartet from Rigoletto. Sadly, Ford later took his life. His loss still brings me sadness. *Oh willow, titwillow, titwillow.*

My first year at Northwestern passed easily, in part because my premedical courses in biochemistry gave me a leg up. However, courses that required memorization, like anatomy, were a challenge. Sometimes I would resort to reason, sometimes the wrong reason.

The brilliant tyrant, Loyal Davis, the Chair of Surgery, taught the freshman fall course in correlative anatomy. The final examination in December or January consisted of a single question:

> *A boy dove into Lake Michigan. When he rose to the surface, he could not move his lower or upper extremities. What caused this?*

This was a simple question with a simple answer:

> *The boy had struck his head, fractured his cervical spine, and transected his cervical spinal cord. In an instant, he had become a quadriplegic… end of story.*

However, consider that winter had come to Chicago. On the surface of Lake Michigan floated cakes of ice. Additionally, the question states that the "*boy rose to the surface.*" Clearly the ice wasn't very thick. When the ice is thick (and it can be very thick) you might as well try diving through cement. The boy would have been on the surface of the Lake. Obviously, the question was posed in a way to see if I realized that the ice was too thin to pose a risk of injury. I took the facts at hand, and gave a simple, possible, but wildly wrong answer: *the boy froze!* I imagine Davis reading my answer and thinking "*God, did this kid learn nothing? He's putting me on!*" Although terribly off the mark, the answer *could* have been correct. If Davis had had a sense of humor, he might have thought my answer was (unintentionally) clever. Davis didn't have a sense of humor. Nevertheless, he gave me a passing grade.

I Decide to Become an Anesthesiologist

My decision to pursue anesthesia as my life's work came suddenly, in a single day (or less), in the summer between my first and second years at Northwestern. Before medical school I envisioned becoming a general practitioner. I had wanted to emulate Dr. Robert Koch, a country physician who had made great medical discoveries, but an epiphany in the operating room changed my mind.

I needed to earn money for my tuition and looked for a paying summer job in some aspect of medicine. *But what job?* Loyal Davis believed anesthesiology unworthy of a Northwestern student's study. That didn't deter about 10 of my classmates from applying for anesthesia externships. They would be preceptees, learn the trade, and be paid to take call for their preceptors. *Yikes!* None of us knew any more of anesthesia than what we had been taught in the first-year course on pharmacology. The audacity and stupidity of that choice makes me tremble today, but the experience sounded interesting, and would help pay the bills. I applied and had the good fortune to be accepted by two anesthesiologists, Lloyd Gittleson and Gwen Gleave. They worked at Grant Hospital in Chicago and happened, I later learned, to be splendid teachers.

I arrived for work on a sunny spring day in 1952, dressed for the operating room, and sat at the head of the operating table on which lay a patient for some minor procedure. Dr. Gittleson inserted a steel needle (no plastic intravenous cannulas then) into a vein and through that infused a dilute solution of thiopental. I was instructed to deliver a combination of oxygen and nitrous oxide to the patient via a black rubber mask I held to the patient's face. The mask was connected by tubing to a circle absorption system that supplied the nitrous oxide and oxygen. A rubber bag attached to the system revealed the patient's breathing in its rhythmical contractions and reexpansions with each breath.

At this juncture, Dr. Gittleson was called from the room. I was left alone to tend to the patient. The thiopental flowed, the bag rhythmically contracted and expanded, and I tightly held the black mask to the patient's face. As seconds passed, the bag moved less and less. It eventually stopped moving altogether. I knew little of anesthesia, or medicine for that matter, but I did know that breathing was good and not breathing was bad. I told the surgeon that the patient had stopped breathing. He would have been within his rights by the standards of that time to have suggested that breathing was my business. Instead he asked if I wanted him to provide artificial ventilation. *"Yes!"*, I said. *"Please!"* He proceeded to intermittently squeeze the chest while the circulating nurse fetched Dr. Gittleson. When he returned, he pointed out that I could have compressed the bag to breathe for the patient. *"It goes both ways, you see?"*

The remainder of the day passed uneventfully. At the day's end, I sat in the locker room slowly dressing, stinking with the sweat of the terror that had stayed with me throughout the day. I thought, *"You could have killed a patient today. And if you decided on a career in anesthesia, you could do that every day…every day take a patient's life in your hands. Every day!"* This was a life changing discovery: anesthesia is power. I responded like a child offered candy. The notion that I would follow the steps of Robert Koch or Ignaz Semmelweis vanished. My new dream was anesthesia, my ticket to money and power!

My career was thus shaped by two epiphanies a decade apart:

1. I didn't want to be a shoe salesman.
2. I wanted to be an anesthesiologist.

I have focused on this career-changing story because of its importance to my life. However, I was motivated by more than a naked desire to have the lives of other humans in my hands. Indeed, a second motive existed, the result of two identical experiences. At age 6 or 7 years I had repeated upper respiratory tract infections that led my pediatrician to prescribe a tonsillectomy and adenoidectomy, duly carried out under ether anesthesia. Anesthesia with ether also followed an accident at age 10 years. For the induction of both anesthetics I was restrained and forced to breathe ether from a facemask. The pungency of the ether made breathing difficult. Superimposed on a sense of strangulation, a black vortex drew me down into a crescendo of buzzing as consciousness disappeared. Each of these two terrifying experiences lasted only moments, but they were moments I wanted never to experience again. By becoming an anesthesiologist, I might discover better drugs to induce anesthesia without the terror.

I became expert in this craft called anesthesia. I read everything I could find concerning anesthesia. I attended the few anesthesia conferences that Chicago had to offer. My studies led to the wonderful finding that there wasn't much to learn other than clinical techniques that promoted smoothness and safety in anesthetic delivery. Wonderful because I might be able to learn everything there might be to know about anesthesia. It was clear that anesthesia was applied pharmacology and physiology, especially respiratory physiology. My patient's brush with death was not a rare possibility. Anesthesia depressed breathing and removed the airway reflexes that protected the awake patient. Breathing and airway problems were common anesthetic problems, and I learned that avoiding these was crucial to the safe conduct of anesthesia. However, I could not find much science that addressed what were clearly problems amenable to study.

The Second and Later Years of Medical School

Now that I was in Northwestern University Medical School, I no longer had to prove myself. I had done that. Initially I could not shrug off my need to succeed at a high level and continued to study to excess. By my second year, I realized:

1. I didn't have to get A's.
2. My peers were an order of magnitude smarter than the students I had competed with at the University of Illinois.

Academically, I excelled that first year and then became an average student. Between the first and succeeding years I had chosen a specialty to pursue. And during this time my mother was dying. I'm not certain I was aware of this or that it affected me. In 1953, she died in our house in the suburbs; my father saddened that he could not help her, could not save her.

Sometime in my second year of medical school, I seized an opportunity that I had eschewed during college where I took course after course devoted to science and mathematics. Northwestern's downtown campus (the medical and law schools) had a liberal arts night school. I signed up, taking courses in Shakespeare, art, and civics. They were wonderful, full of delights that I had missed in college and not appreciated when taught in high school. *Yes, even civics!* I learned there is more to life than studying, and more to knowledge than science.

I have always been timid. I still am. In my fourth year in medical school I assisted in the repair of a hernia in a 6-year-old boy. I held a retractor. The operation proceeded under open-drop ether anesthesia delivered by a resident supervised by an attending anesthesiologist. By now I had learned enough to know that the patient's stertorous breathing indicated airway obstruction. I longed for the airway to be cleared. Gagged by traditions (medical students don't correct residents; surgeons don't manage anesthesia) I said nothing. The child suffered a respiratory arrest, followed by cardiovascular collapse and death. *Would anyone have listened had I spoken up? Probably not.* Nevertheless, I still blame myself for not speaking, for being timid, for being intimidated by artificial boundaries and stupid traditions.

Loyal Davis Does Me a Favor

Students always make fun of the faculty, and we were no exception. Dr. Davis was a particularly good target. We served in the home delivery (maternity) service and were occasionally consulted by impoverished mothers of newborn black children on recommendations for names. Mothers occasionally accepted our recommendation for the name "Loyal Davis" Jones. Sometimes we were found out. Anxious that Dr. Davis would torpedo our medical careers, we urgently tracked down the parents and implored them to choose another name lest we be denied permission to graduate. Despite his sometimes tyranny, I admired Davis as a brilliant teacher who was not arbitrary in his tyranny. I also respected his intelligence. Every year he invited the new medical students to his home. After introducing himself to each one, he then escorted his wife around the room and introduced each new student by name.

In my senior year, Loyal Davis interviewed me, as he did all students nearing graduation. My father had not been impressed with my choice of anesthesia as a career, and Dr. Davis shared his disdain for the profession. He did not believe anesthesia merited the talents of a male Northwestern graduate. As I entered his office, he shook his finger at me and said, *"You're a smart aleck."* Perhaps he had remembered my answer to why the boy who dove into Lake Michigan had become paralyzed. Davis never explained his comment to me.

The interview followed. Davis asked if I knew of the concerns that had recently risen in the specialty of Anesthesiology regarding the form by which anesthesiologists were compensated for their services: *salary or fee for service?* I did not. He then said that I would write an essay concerning the ethics of each approach to compensation and that the essay would be completed to his satisfaction before I graduated. By this he did me a favor, forcing me to interview several anesthesiologists including the great Henry Beecher.

Months after I submitted my report, I met Davis on the street and asked him if he'd liked the essay. He hadn't read it. I graduated anyway.

Internship and Residency

4

I Marry Dollie Ross

As mentioned in the last chapter, I'm a timid man. If the Queen knights me, I will choose the title Sir Ted the Timid. In my third year of medical school, I courted Dollie Ross (**Figure 4.1**), a Northwestern student of speech therapy. It took 2 years for me to gather sufficient courage to ask her to marry me. She said yes! *Huzzah!* Just after graduation, on June 15, 1955, we married. My father was my best man. For several years, Dollie and I shared a close and happy life.

Internship

I interned at St. Luke's Hospital in Chicago, a rotating internship that broadened my clinical experience and gave me time to seek a good residency. Dad gave us the keys to one of several apartments he owned near Wrigley Field, which would be our housing for the year of my internship. Midway through internship St. Luke's generously doubled my starting salary of $25 per month. Although it still wasn't much money, housing, uniforms, and food were free. My father partially underwrote our living expenses and Dollie became a speech therapist, thereby providing additional financial support.

Choosing a Residency

I had no organized approach to choosing a residency. I visited Midwest programs, and one distinguished program in Boston. The prestigious program in Boston had nothing but unhappy residents. They uniformly advised me to go elsewhere. Eventually I chose the University of Iowa. In medical school, I had become an avid reader of everything I could find about the practice of anesthesia. One of my treasures was Stuart Cullen's *Anesthesia in General Practice*, a booklet of 200 pages that went through numerous editions. I still have a partial collection of six editions. Dr. Cullen was the head of the anesthesia program at the University of Iowa. Based on his book, I applied for a residency at the University of Iowa. When I visited, Dr. Cullen invited me to stay at his house. The book, the outstanding program, and the courtesy extended by Dr. Cullen led me to choose the University of Iowa. I don't think I could have done better.

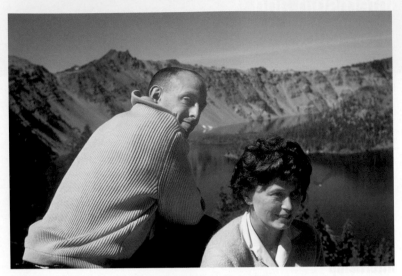

Figure 4.1 Dollie and me at Crater Lake Oregon in the early 1960s.

Early one July day in 1956, 16 fellow residents and I arrived for our indoctrination into the 2-year anesthesia program at the University of Iowa. Residency at that time was vastly different from today's training. For example, I was on call the first evening of residency... my first day as a resident! I didn't know a great deal but from my attention to anesthesia as an extern in medical school and subsequent studies, I knew more than most of my fellow residents. I called Dollie to ask for toiletries and clean underwear. Emergency cases had already been listed. For my first case, I would anesthetize a farmer's wife who had an empyematous gall bladder. All the faculty had left for the comforts of home and dinner. I wasn't exactly on my own. There was a team "leader," a newly minted second-year resident. I asked for guidance: "What should I do?" He suggested an epidural anesthetic and showed me how. The rest of the evening was a blur. I quickly learned to give an epidural anesthetic. My patients and I survived.

Residency Supervision in the 1950s

My first official day in anesthesia illustrates the limited supervision of residents at the time. This unfortunate necessity reflected the short supply of trained anesthesiologists. Anesthesia was not the prized specialty that it is today. Since they were in short supply, a single faculty member might supply the supervision of three, four, or five residents independently conducting as many cases at a given time during the day. Faculty disappeared to home in the evenings. They were on call, but rarely were called. I remember calling my faculty only twice during my 2 years of training. For one, I had been asked to see a young housewife who was comatose from some unknown evil that had devastated her brain. I was asked for suggestions for her management and could think of none, so I called Bill Hamilton. To his credit he soon appeared at the hospital (I didn't ask him to come). Unfortunately, Dr. Hamilton was similarly perplexed. The patient died despite our efforts.

One evening, later in my residency, I was assigned to provide anesthesia for a newborn afflicted with a tracheoesophageal fistula. Having never dealt with such a problem I called my consultant, Dr. Cullen, who advised intubation of the trachea and controlled ventilation by hand. I followed his directions, not expecting further guidance. About 20 minutes later Dr. Cullen was at my side, saying little, yet guiding (or was it overseeing?) my every move.

I Learn the Correct Dose of Phenylephrine

I hadn't been at Iowa more than a few weeks when I was assigned a list of cases in the cystoscopy suite. The primary procedures were transurethral prostatectomies and transurethral removal of bladder tumors. We used a spinal anesthetic with procaine for such procedures. Why procaine? "Because anesthesia wouldn't last more than an hour." The brief time course of procaine spinal anesthesia mitigated the risk of the absorbing too much irrigation fluid. Roughly 45 minutes after injection of the procaine, the patient would terminate the procedure with a well-placed kick.

The fourth-floor cystoscopy suite lay two floors below the main operating suite. Like all residents, I took my drugs and equipment with me. I kept everything I might need in a carpenter's toolbox. We usually were unsupervised in the urology suite. "If you need help, call upstairs."

I had performed few spinal anesthetics previously, but I'd read how to do it. I felt ready. My first patient was a genial Iowa farmer. Insertion of the spinal needle and injection of 100 mg of procaine went without incident. Clearly, I was getting better at this anesthesia thing. But then, the blood pressure decreased, as it will with spinal anesthesia. "No problem" I thought, "I'll just give a vasopressor." I rummaged in my toolbox, finding a 10-mg ampule of phenylephrine. "Let's see. How much should I give?" I reasoned that an ampule would contain a standard dose, but I cautiously gave just a quarter of the contents of the ampule. The farmer soon looked up at me saying, "Doc, I have a terrible headache." His normal blood pressure of 120/80 mm Hg had risen to over 300 mm Hg. That was as great a pressure as my sphygmomanometer displayed. I had the wit not to do more than wait, and the hypertension and headache resolved in a matter of minutes. I had learned more about the standard dose of phenylephrine than any text could teach me. I've not forgotten. 2.5 mg of phenylephrine is too much.

Learning From My Errors

One aspect of residency that hasn't changed is that we learn to give anesthesia from our errors as well as from direct instruction by faculty and reading. Providing anesthesia stressed all of us. We truly did (and do) have the patient's life in our hands at every moment. Weariness at the day's end limited our learning by reading.

Dr. Cullen was kind and forgiving. We revered him for his honesty and openness to contradiction. We knew we could say anything, oppose anything, share any thought, without fear that we would offend him. Even today as I write this, I think of him as Dr. Cullen. A few (never I) called him "Stu." Dr. Cullen eventually bought a vanity license plate saying, "Stu who?" However, even today, most of us wouldn't call him anything other than Dr. Cullen.

I remained intensely curious. Having no concern for what the Institutional Review Board (IRB) might say (IRBs didn't exist), I was free to try this or that, and I did. I'd read about the use of intramuscular injection of succinylcholine to produce the paralysis that might facilitate tracheal intubation, and I applied it with abandon. One morning, absent faculty in my operating room in the Ear, Nose and Throat suite, I anesthetized an infant with a cleft lip and palate with ether. The infant sustained his airway and breathed spontaneously. Then I gave an intramuscular injection of succinylcholine. As I had anticipated, paralysis followed the injection. I had not anticipated that despite my best efforts I could neither intubate the trachea nor ventilate the lungs by application of positive pressure with a mask. Now terrified, I called for my faculty supervisor, Dr. Jack Moyers, who quickly arrived. Dr. Moyers found that he, too, could neither intubate the trachea nor ventilate the lungs, at least initially. With great effort, he finally placed the tracheal tube and the crisis passed. Then, learning what I had done, he (correctly) called me an idiot and other things that Dr. Cullen would not have called me.

I've wondered if the faculty considered firing me for the freedoms I took with patients and equipment. They seemed to support my forays into research, but that didn't mean they approved of my liberties with common sense. So many years later (in September 2014), I asked Bill Hamilton if I had been at risk of being fired. He assured me that the question of my employment had never been raised. But then he added, "Of course I'm 92 now and my memory may be faulty."

When pressed to supply further details, Bill commented kindly but with few specifics:

First, you were always dependable. You came to work, remained at work etc. You were polite and respectful to those with whom you and the Department had frequent work contact. It was done well.

Second, you were appropriate as a resident. I never recall your creating an angry surgeon. You didn't create an atmosphere in which surgeons felt they were losing control of their patient and MOST importantly you did not threaten the surgeon as to his proper status in the Operating Room or elsewhere in the hospital world.

Third, you always did at least your share of the workload. You were not one who shifted tasks to others...I do not recall any social or personal behavior that was inflammatory or derogatory to patients, instructors, nurses etc...I have not noted dishonesty in any of your social contacts...

Lastly, you didn't support the Iowa Hawkeyes with the enthusiasm that I do. Despite that inexplicable behavior flaw I believe you to have a respectable social conscience...I see you as an example of the broadly-based knowledge I feel we should all try for.

I Was Drawn to Research as a Resident

The faculty at Iowa supported research activities by residents. My curiosity led from one-off experiments with patients under my care to formal studies. With Bill Hamilton, I devised a simple device with no moving parts that could supply positive-negative pressure ventilation[1] at a time when negative intratracheal pressure was thought to be potentially advantageous because it might support the circulation by drawing blood back into the lungs. But a negative pressure could cause pulmonary collapse, and no one ever took up my wonderful device.

Hugh Keasling in the Department of Pharmacology and I studied meprobamate versus pentobarbital versus nothing as premedications in adults. We found that meprobamate or pentobarbital given before bedtime, and repeated before surgery, increased sleep and decreased anxiety in young patients, but not in old or senile patients.[2] These are not surprising findings, but they did guide patient care.

In my last year of residency, again with Bill Hamilton's help, I made my first real foray into pharmacology. Brodie and colleagues had shown that reserpine, a drug used clinically to treat hypertension, caused the depletion of intracellular catecholamines.[3] An earlier study by Gaddum and Kwiatkowski suggested ephedrine might act by inhibiting the metabolism of catecholamines,[4] increasing the clinical effect of endogenously released catecholamines. Based on their hypothesized mechanism of action, we predicted reserpine might limit the pressor action of ephedrine and similar compounds.[5]

We found that prior reserpine treatment indeed interfered with the physiological effects of ephedrine. Dogs given reserpine had almost no increase in blood pressure and heart rate following administration of ephedrine or other vasopressors (eg, amphetamines) that acted by indirectly increasing the concentration of circulating catecholamines. However, vasopressors that directly acted on blood vessels and the heart (eg, epinephrine and phenylephrine) continued to be effective after reserpine treatment. Fortunately, we recognized that there were several explanations for our observations, concluding that "speculation on the relation between amine oxidase inhibiting properties of ephedrine and methamphetamine (and mephentermine) or other enzyme inhibiting properties and their consequent impotency following reserpine injection cannot be supported or denied by the above experiment." That proved prescient, because the mechanism proposed by Gaddum and Kwiatkowski was eventually proven wrong. Although the mechanism is still not entirely known, ephedrine does not work by inhibiting metabolism of catecholamines. The mechanism of action is some combination of facilitation of the release of stored catecholamines from nerve terminals and direction action on adrenergic receptors.[6,7]

Residents at Iowa Gave Lectures, and One Changed My Life

Iowa anesthesiology residents were expected to contribute lectures. One of my lectures was a tutorial on non-rebreathing systems, particularly Ayre's T-piece. This is an anesthetic delivery system that fascinated me. I was certain that it would similarly fascinate the residents and faculty. At the end of my presentation, Bill Hamilton assured me that I had given one of the dullest lectures of the year. "Perhaps several years," he added.

Not all resident lectures were dull. We had a new resident, John Severinghaus, who came from another anesthesia residency program (the University of Pennsylvania). He had taken his first year of residency in 1952 but was drafted for service from 1953 to 1956. In 1954, while in the service, he reported on the uptake of nitrous oxide in humans, work he had done while a resident in Philadelphia.[8] This elegant research was the first measurement of the uptake of any inhaled anesthetic in humans or animals, other than Haggard's earlier work in the 1920s with ether in dogs.[9,10] In 1956, John came to Iowa to complete his second year of residency.

But I digress. Lecturing in 1956 as a resident at Iowa, John described his simple study, putting it in the context of what then was known about the factors governing the uptake and distribution of inhaled anesthetics. John propounded the astonishing notion that the effect of more soluble anesthetics would develop more slowly than the effect of less soluble anesthetics. Being the smart aleck that Loyal Davis had recognized in me, and not appreciating the genius that John was, I argued against this notion. "More of a more soluble anesthetic will be taken up, and thus more will get to the brain than with a less soluble anesthetic. If more gets to the brain, shouldn't that accelerate the effect?" "No", said John. The argument continued well after the lecture ended. We concluded the dispute that night with each certain that the other was wrong. But only one of us could be right. John was. He almost always was.

John's lecture changed my life. Guided by imagination, physiology, anatomy, and the little that had been written about uptake and distribution, I increasingly thought about the factors that governed uptake and distribution, this movement of inhaled anesthetics into, within, and out of the body. The great Seymour Kety had proposed one scheme,[11] but he failed to recognize the importance of the differential distribution of blood flow. Additionally, Kety's complex mathematical scheme could not be understood by most mortals. Blood flow differs among tissues, being greater to brain than muscle, and greater to muscle than fat. A correct scheme describing uptake and distribution must account for the influence of differential flow in how much these tissues take up anesthetics. Henry Price took differential blood flow into account in his later description of the uptake and distribution of thiopental.[12] But Price's scheme did not account for the ventilatory factors inherent in a description of the uptake and distribution of inhaled anesthetics.

We Have Our First Child

The birth of our first child, Cris Cadence, at the end of my first year of residency changed my personal life forever. Among many purchases, we bought a sturdy second-hand Iowa oak rocking chair that I used to rock Cris and three subsequent Eger children. We fed them, sang to them, and rocked them in that chair until they fell asleep. Sometimes we fell asleep concurrently and the rocking stopped. Cris still has the chair.

We moved. Cris's entry into the world entitled us to occupy low-cost student housing. We shared a 24-by-40-foot Quonset hut with another student family, and numerous roaches that were included with the residence. Ridding ourselves of the roaches required coordinated spraying of insecticide; otherwise the bugs avoided death by shuttling from one to the other side of the Quonset hut.

Apple Pie and the Berry Plan

During my internship, my father partially underwrote our living expenses. Dollie worked as a speech therapist to further supplement our income. Fortunately, during residency, my salary increased to a living, if not generous, wage. Dollie and I had achieved financial independence. Our Quonset hut student housing helped further. And although Dollie no longer worked as a speech therapist, she made ends meet in various ways. One dinner ended with apple pie, or so I thought. Dollie asked if I had liked the desert, and I enthusiastically said yes. She then revealed that the apple pie had been made with soda crackers and a pinch of cinnamon. No apples. Wives can be amazing.

I finished my residency in 1958, fascinated by the concepts bubbling in my mind about uptake and distribution. To allow me to complete my residency before induction into the armed services, I enlisted in the US Army under the terms of the Berry Plan. This required that I serve in the Army for 2 years following residency. In July, I began to fulfill that obligation, not realizing that it would provide an unexpected opportunity to develop and test my ideas about uptake and distribution.

References

1. Eger EI, Hamilton WK. Positive-negative pressure ventilation with a modified Ayre's T-piece. *Anesthesiology*. 1958;19:611-618.
2. Eger EI II, Keasling HH. Comparison of meprobamate, pentobarbital, and placebo as preanesthetic medication for regional procedures. *Anesthesiology*. 1959;20:1-9.
3. Brodie BB, Olin JS, Kuntzman RG, Shore PA. Possible interrelationship between release of brain norepinephrine and serotonin by reserpine. *Science*. 1957;125:1293-1294.
4. Gaddum JH, Kwiatkowski H. The action of ephedrine. *J Physiol*. 1938;94:87-100.
5. Eger EI II, Hamilton WK. The effect of reserpine on the action of various vasopressors. *Anesthesiology*. 1959;20:641-645.
6. Kobayashi S, Endou M, Sakuraya F, et al. The sympathomimetic actions of l-ephedrine and d-pseudoephedrine: direct receptor activation or norepinephrine release? *Anesth Analg*. 2003;97:1239-1245.
7. Liles JT, Dabisch PA, Hude KE, et al. Pressor responses to ephedrine are mediated by a direct mechanism in the rat. *J Pharmacol Exp Ther*. 2006;316:95-105.
8. Severinghaus JW. The rate of uptake of nitrous oxide in man. *J Clin Invest*. 1954;33:1183-1189.
9. Haggard AW. The absorption, distribution and elimination of ethyl ether. II. Analysis of the mechanism of absorption and elimination of such a gas or vapor as ethyl ether. *J Biol Chem*. 1924;59:753-796.
10. Haggard AW. The absorption, distribution and elimination of ethyl ether. III. The relation of the concentration of ether, or any similar volatile substance in the central nervous system to the concentration in the arterial blood and the buffer action of the body. *J Biol Chem*. 1924;59:797-832.
11. Kety SS. Theory and application of exchange of inert gas at the lungs and tissues. *Pharmacol Rev*. 1951;3:1-41.
12. Price HL. A dynamic concept of the distribution of thiopental in the human body. *Anesthesiology*. 1960;21:40-5.

Fort Leavenworth, Kansas

5

Indoctrination and Posting in the US Army

I spent my first 6 weeks in the Army at Fort Sam Houston in San Antonio, Texas. Fort Sam Houston is a dry and dusty military base that nonetheless was a pleasant introduction to Army service. I set about learning duties, obligations, opportunities, and traditions. With dozens of other drafted physicians, I learned to salute, fire a rifle, wear a gas mask, squirm under machine gun fire, and march (but not too far). One day, my peers and I assembled for a several-mile parade. We set off in formation, walking at a comfortable pace. I glanced back, noting that an ambulance followed us, apparently in anticipation of some fallouts. The Army was smarter than I had anticipated. Indeed, initial expectations to the contrary (for no good reason), my orders and instructions all seemed quite rational.

We graduated from orientation and were asked where we might like to be posted. This was a kind, considerate, but entirely meaningless gesture. I said either the East or West coast would be fine. The Army compromised, stationing me at Fort Leavenworth, Kansas.

My Good Fortune!

Fort Leavenworth is near the town of Leavenworth, Kansas. The military base and the town are home to several penitentiaries, including two military prisons at Fort Leavenworth, and the infamous United States Penitentiary in the city of Leavenworth. Given this abundance, I thought I might spend my time tending to the medical needs of prisoners. I did tend to prisoners. However, more commonly I anesthetized majors, colonels, and generals, none of whom were imprisoned at the time.

Fort Leavenworth is home to the United States Army Command and General Staff College. As an elite military graduate school, Fort amenities included a 27-hole golf course. It seemed that everyone on the base was an officer. As an Army Captain, I was among the lower ranking officers.

I was paged on arriving at the post. Good grief, *who knew I was here?* Colonel Boyson, the senior surgeon, ordered me to the obstetrical ward.

Would I please insert an IV needle in this patient whose veins had defied Colonel Boyson? Of course! I was off to a good start! After inserting the IV, I went to the administrative office to complete the formalities needed to work at the hospital. The master sergeant in charge asked if there were anything he might help me with. *"Did I need a second car?"* I did, and he had one to sell, a vintage Packard, for $50. *How could I go wrong?* After buying it, I found that it had holes in the floor, providing natural air conditioning. But it was a heavy car with rear wheel drive undaunted by Kansas snow and ice. Two years later I sold it for $100. My early lessons in capitalism from catching flies were proving useful.

What I Did

I had a grand title: Chief of the Anesthesia and Operative Section. As such I directed the activities in two operating rooms. One was of normal size, but the other was slightly bigger than a closet. With the help of two nurse anesthetists, I supplied anesthesia for each. Both anesthetists were competent. Indeed, Major Idelle Kraft was a superb clinician. Although my title was Chief of the Anesthesia and Operative Section, the real boss was the NCO (Non-Commissioned Officer) for the operating area, Master Sergeant Bufford. He guided me through a successful 2-year career.

On matters of importance I would ask for and follow Sergeant Bufford's advice. I remember failing to ask for his advice, on a sensitive subject. It proved to be a big mistake. Despite his problems with starting IVs, Col. Boyson was a competent surgeon with one flaw. He regularly arrived late for his surgeries. The nurses would be ready, and I'd have the patient anesthetized, and then we would wait. Without consulting Sergeant Bufford, after one particularly long wait, I gently suggested to the Colonel that he please arrive on time. Col. Boyson had been a tank commander in World War II. In full tank commander voice, he told me that if I ever made that suggestion again he would see to it that I was reassigned to Korea. I never repeated the suggestion.

I usually finished work at noon. Occasionally, I had other duties such as giving officers physical examinations. I remember finding a lump in an officer's thyroid one afternoon and anesthetizing him the next day for removal of his cancer. But most afternoons I could do as I pleased. I tried the 27-hole golf course but found that it held little attraction for me. My skill in golf hadn't improved since my youth.

Leavenworth and Ft. Leavenworth were pleasant places, enhanced by their proximity to Kansas City, a reasonably large metropolis. I attended the weekly seminars at the Department of Anesthesiology at the University of Kansas, developing an affection for the Department. I thought to return there if they would have me when I finished my career in the Army. It never happened. Instead, I was seduced by life at the University of California, described in Chapter 6.

Dollie and I lived in the town of Leavenworth for our first year in the Army. In our second year, we moved to Fort Leavenworth. Next door were our friends, the Bookers, he a carpenter and she a housewife. Each Sunday Cris Booker and I would walk to the corner store for supplies and the Sunday paper, accompanied along the way by a neighbor's large black Labrador.

Fortunately, golf was not the only entertainment option provided by the Army. Dollie and I tried playing duplicate bridge, but our second or third experience dissuaded us from persisting. I was dealt an oddly fortuitous hand with seven cards of one suit. We made an extravagant bid, which we won. Our opponents were Vivian and Hank Krawchek. Hank was a radiologist. Vivian did not take well to losing. She upbraided me, fuming "*You should not have bid so much! You had no right to make the bid!*" We apologized but kept our winning score. I thought I saw her husband smile.

We availed ourselves of theater in Kansas City, once coming a week late to a performance of The Music Man. The theater took mercy on us, giving us left over seats in the balcony.

Dollie bore a second child, Doreen Joyce Eger, so now we were four and the rocking chair did double duty. Dori began to walk 9 months after birth, but her walking was peculiar. "*She walks like a little old woman*," said Dollie. Dori had a congenitally dislocated hip that the pediatrician, Major Joernes, had overlooked at birth. For a year, Dori wore a cast that slowly caused the restructuring of that hip to normal. I made devices that accommodated her cast and allowed her to sit up and to be mobile. She could scoot along at great speed, but she was not happy with her confinement in a plaster cast.

Most of our time was spent raising our children. We read stories and sang to them in that heavy Iowa rocking chair. We took family vacations to Sioux Falls to visit Dollie's parents, or to Chicago to visit my parents. I busied myself with writing equations in the attic of the hospital, giving anesthesia or physical examinations, reading, sleeping, and eating. My days passed easily in my thoroughly unremarkable life at Fort Leavenworth. Without realizing it at the time, I was setting the foundation for my life's work. It's easier to judge life through the rear-view mirror than through the windshield.

The Blue Patient

I continued to experiment with my patients. No Institutional Review Board (IRB) existed to advise me otherwise. I had the notion that positive pressure ventilation should cause the extravascular movement of intravascular fluid, thereby decreasing intravascular fluid volume. I consulted with my friends in the clinical laboratory and found that they could determine intravascular fluid volume by injecting Evans Blue dye intravenously and measuring the resulting blood concentration of the dye. Evans Blue, I read, was a harmless substance that disappeared from the body. One of the patients in the prisoners' ward was to have an orthopedic procedure that required my care. I took the opportunity, while he was anesthetized, to inject Evans Blue to measure his blood volume with and without positive pressure ventilation.

I don't remember how many times I repeated the injection during his procedure to make the measurement, but it was many times. By the end of the procedure, the prisoner turned a dusky blue. I had anticipated this possibility but understood that the color change was short-lived. It was not. Perhaps a month later, toward the end of November, the physician in charge of the hospital, a dermatologist, stopped me in the hospital hallway. *"Dr. Eger,"* he said. *"Would you please do me a favor?"* "Yes, sir", I replied, *"What might that be?"* "I'd like you to turn that patient in the orthopedic ward back to a normal color by Thanksgiving." The color did fade with time. A long time. My one-off, one-patient study with Evans Blue (I never did that again) wasn't a stellar contribution to research.

More Successful Research

I had better luck with other studies. One made use of Major Kraft's talents. She managed the anesthesia for tonsillectomies and adenoidectomies, anesthetizing all these pediatric patients with the same divinyl-ether/diethyl-ether sequence. Same procedure, same anesthetic, same superb anesthetist. It allowed for a controlled comparison of the effect of differences in premedication. As we said in the opening statement of the report that resulted: "Approaches to the problem of preanesthetic medication in children are infinite as may be inferred from the variety of drugs and dose schedules advocated. Few controlled studies have been done and these have failed to show any great differences in the effectiveness of any particular drug or drug combination."[1] That was about to change.

In our double-blinded, randomized study of 248 children,[1] we gave vagolytic agents (atropine or scopolamine) with either nothing (the control), an opioid (morphine or meperidine), or with a barbiturate (pentobarbital) as premedication. Those given scopolamine had less fretfulness and irritability, reduced secretions, and more drowsiness than those given atropine (**Table 5.1**). The addition of an opioid or barbiturate added several other significant ($P < 0.01$) differences. Most impressive to me were

Table 5.1 Study Showing Opioid Premedication Increases Postoperative Nausea and Vomiting in Children[1]

		Comparison Between Premedicants and Factors Statistically Significant			
Factor	Age Group	Vagolytic Alone	Meperidine + Vagolytic	Morphine + Vagolytic	Pentobarbital + Vagolytic
Time to intubation (minutes)*	Both	11.35	11.22	9.04	9.98
Active preanesthetic cooperation* Uncooperative (%)	5 & younger	29	12	36	45
Decrease in fretfulness and irritability (%)	5 & younger*	26	48	61	30
	6 & older	32	33	48	50
Minimal second stage excitement (%)*	Both	63	76	82	82
Minimal mucous secretion during induction (%)†	Both	52	78	85	57
Smooth induction (%)*	Both	56	65	79	61
Minimal laryngospasm (%)*	Both	73	87	94	82
Minimal mucous secretion during maintenance (%)*	Both	61	82	77	67

(Continued)

Table 5.1 Study Showing Opioid Premedication Increases Postoperative Nausea and Vomiting in Children[1]   (Continued)

		Comparison Between Premedicants and Factors Statistically Significant			
Factor	Age Group	Vagolytic Alone	Meperidine + Vagolytic	Morphine + Vagolytic	Pentobarbital + Vagolytic
Not perspiring (%)†	Both	79	61	81	90
Excited in the recovery room (%)†	Both	34	17	9	26
Vomiting (%)†	Both	39	71	71	18
Moderate-marked vomiting (%)*	Both	16	38	33	0
Judged adequately premedicated (%)†	Both	76	90	98	83

*P < 0.05.
†P < 0.01.

the differences in postoperative vomiting. 39% of control patients vomited, but only 18% of patients given pentobarbital vomited. However, a whopping 71% of patients given an opioid vomited. It didn't matter whether the opioid was morphine or meperidine; 71% in each group vomited. Today we might explain these differences by effects on opioid and $GABA_A$ receptors.

In another study, I showed that high inflow rates of nitrous oxide were necessary to rapidly change alveolar anesthetic concentration.[2] It seemed important at the time, but in retrospect seems obvious, even trivial.

Solving Equations by Iteration

The three-story wood-and-brick Army hospital was many decades old. Our quarters, complete with gigantic cockroaches, bordered the hospital. I had to walk but 100 ft and pass an enormous ginkgo tree to arrive at my operating room. I remember it as the loveliest of trees.

No one seemed interested in the hospital's third floor except me. It became my cavernous office, requiring only a desk, chair, and light. Each afternoon I retreated to it. Over my 2 years of service in the Army, I developed simple iterative equations that described my vision of the movement of anesthetic molecules into and out of the body.[3] Each respiration constituted a cycle, and within each cycle, anesthetic moved as a step change from inspired gas to lung to blood to individual tissues.

Writing the equations did not complete the answer. The equations had to be solved to describe the time course of the resulting concentrations in the lungs and tissues. And the solutions had to produce results consistent with actual data, to be reasonable approximations to the truth.

Solving the equations presented two problems. The solutions were iterative, repeated hundreds of times to generate a curve describing the result of 50 minutes of anesthesia. Today this would be a trivial task, child's play for a computer. But I had no computer. I did have a gigantic slide rule, accurate to four places. I still have it. But four places would not provide sufficient accuracy, because errors could add up over many iterations. My calculations required a mechanical calculator. Fortune smiled. The dietitian for the hospital had a clunky mechanical calculator accurate to 16 places. I have no idea why she needed a calculator accurate to 16 places. She let me use it in the afternoons. Even with this calculator, it took the better part of 2 days to calculate concentration changes for 50 minutes of anesthesia. That seems slow now but was a breakthrough at the time.

I needed to compare my predictions to actual clinical data. My small hospital had no access to grand research equipment. No problem! For clinical care I had a modern polarographic oxygen sensor to measure dissolved oxygen concentration to an accuracy of 1%. I could analyze the nitrous oxide concentration in a mixture of oxygen and nitrous oxide if I knew the concentration of oxygen and had eliminated all of the nitrogen. And so I did.

My mathematical solution employed a simplification. I assumed that the gas space into which I delivered nitrous oxide immediately mixed with the gases within that space. I approximated this assumption in my patient studies by hyperventilating the lungs, rapidly mixing the gas in the patient's lungs with the gas in the anesthetic circuit. My predicted concentrations closely matched my measured concentrations.[4]

I Didn't Believe the Results

The equations made a prediction I had not anticipated. They showed that the inspired concentration of anesthetic influenced the rate at which the alveolar concentration would rise. Of course, giving a greater inspired concentration would increase the absolute alveolar concentration, but the equations went beyond that, finding that a greater inspired concentration would accelerate the *rate* of rise.

This is not obvious, so it may help to work through the example in **Figure 5.1**. In the first vertical bar, the lungs are filled with 1% sevoflurane, 19% oxygen (not optimal, but it makes the math easier), and 80% nitrous oxide. Let this be the first breath during anesthesia. Hold that breath! Over the course of a few seconds, very little oxygen and sevoflurane concentrations will be taken up, but nitrous oxide will be rapidly taken up by the blood. The result is that oxygen and sevoflurane concentrations will rise, rather than fall, as shown is the second vertical bar in **Figure 5.1**. Let's say (again, mostly to make the math easier) that half of the nitrous oxide is absorbed while the breath is being held. This will reduce the lung volume by 40%. With the reduction in lung volume, the concentration of the oxygen will *rise* to 32%, and the concentration of sevoflurane will *rise* to 1.7%. No oxygen or sevoflurane has entered the lungs. Instead, the rapid uptake of nitrous oxide has concentrated the remaining gases.

Now take a breath of the same anesthetic mixture to fill the lungs back to their original volume. The inspired gas is the "added gas" in the third column of **Figure 5.1**. The added gases are in the same proportion of the gases in the first column (1% sevoflurane, 19% oxygen, 80% nitrous oxide), but in **Figure 5.1**, they are labeled as a percent of total lung volume to make the math easier. The oxygen and sevoflurane represented in the second column remain in the lungs, but since the lungs have refilled to their original volume, they have reverted to 19% and 1%, respectively. Because the percentages shown in column 3 are percentages of the final volume, the absolute percentage of each gas can be determined by simply adding the contributions of the original gas with the contributions of the added gas: 27% oxygen, 1.4% sevoflurane, and 72% nitrous oxide.

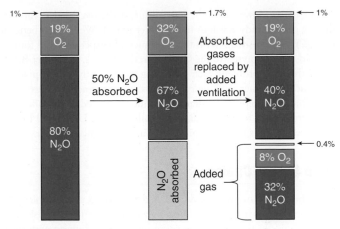

Figure 5.1 The second gas effect.

Figure 5.1 is how we teach this concept today. Separating the effects of concentrating the gases (column 1 to column 2) and the effects of inhaling additional gases (column 2 to column 3) makes the concept reasonably straightforward. However, sitting in the third floor of the Army hospital at Fort Leavenworth, all I knew was that my equations predicted something I did not understand. I had naively assumed that if 10% of an inspired gas yielded an alveolar concentration of 5% in X minutes, 40% of an inspired gas would yield an alveolar concentration of 20% in X minutes as well. However, my equations predicted that a four-fold increase in inspired concentration would produce a four-fold increase in alveolar concentration in fewer than X minutes. I called this effect of the inspired concentration the "concentration effect."[5] I remember initially not believing that the concentration effect existed. But repeating the calculations kept producing the same result. For several years, I simply did not believe the finding, despite the mathematical confirmation and subsequent clinical validation. Eventually I understood the physiology as explained above for **Figure 5.1**. It was only then that I accepted the findings.

I Am Ordered to Wear Dress Blues

The surgeon-general scheduled a visit to the post toward the end of my tour of duty. All medical officers were ordered (*not asked!*) to attend a dress blues reception for the general. That presented a problem. On induction, we were given a uniform allowance of $300 to cover our uniform needs. This allowance nominally covered dress blues. We Berry Plan draftees saw little need to purchase a fancy uniform that we might never wear. Most of us used the money for other purposes. Now we had to have dress blues or face court martial. The $300 was long gone. Frantically, I wrote to one of my regular army buddies posted at Fitzsimmons Army Medical Center in Denver, asking if I could borrow his dress blues. *Of course!* The uniform came just in time. However, at the last minute I discovered that the uniform didn't fit. My good buddy was four inches taller than I. Well, it was better that it was too large than too small. With the assistance of suspenders and four under-shirts, I could present myself to the General in dress blues. The other Berry Plan draftees had the same problem, each managing it differently. Ben Laprade bit the bullet, bought dress blues, and added calling cards—formal business cards. The weekend before the reception he drank too much. Dressed in his fancy uniform he marched from door to door passing out calling cards. Dollie and I drank too much at the reception. Our third child, Ed, was born 9 months later.

Making a Career Choice

Coming to the end of my tour of duty, I had to make a career choice. When I decided on anesthesia, I had done so for money and power. I had envisioned going into private practice in the Midwest, earning money as a clinician with the power over a patient's life inherent in the practice of clinical anesthesia. But during a walk on a beach in Miami, Bill Hamilton told me I showed a talent for academic med-icine. I was captivated by my work on inhaled anesthetic kinetics. I had devised the basics for an understanding of uptake and distribution. I wanted to explore the broader implications of the mathematics that I had developed at Fort Leavenworth. I needed someone to guide me, test me, and inspire me for a year or so while I solved the remaining problems. The answer was obviously to sit at John Severinghaus' feet for that time. John had become Director of Anesthesia Research at the University of California in San Francisco (UCSF). Stuart Cullen had become the Chair of the UCSF Department of Anesthesia. Dollie and I had never been to San Francisco. It seemed like an exciting new adventure for us. I applied and became a trainee starting in July 1960. I thought we would be there for a year or two, completing my studies before I entered private practice. The year became a lifetime.

References

1. Eger EI II, Kraft ID, Keasling HH. A comparison of atropine, or scopolamine, plus pentobarbital, meperidine, or morphine as pediatric preanesthetic medication. *Anesthesiology*. 1961;22:962-969.
2. Eger EI II. Factors affecting the rapidity of alteration of nitrous oxide concentration in a circle system. *Anesthesiology*. 1960;21:348-355.
3. Eger EI II. A mathematical model of uptake and distribution. In: Papper EM, Kitz RJ, eds. *Uptake and Distribution of Anesthetic Agents*. McGraw-Hill; 1963:72-87.
4. Merkel G, Eger EI II. A comparative study of halothane and halopropane anesthesia including method for determining equipotency. *Anesthesiology*. 1963;24:346-357.
5. Eger EI II. The effect of inspired concentration on the rate of rise of alveolar concentration. *Anesthesiology*. 1963;24:153-157.

John Severinghaus

As John's fellow, I quickly learned a few things about him. First, John Severinghaus was creative. He demonstrated that with his elegant simple experiment measuring the uptake of nitrous oxide,[1] and with his development of blood-gas electrode systems. I had watched him do part of that development while he and I were residents at Iowa. Second, John knew more about uptake and distribution than anyone else. Third, he could make any electronic gadget work, exposing me to the workings of infrared analyzers[2] and other devices. Finally, I had wrongly assumed that John was as fascinated with uptake and distribution as I was. Not so. John's passion was understanding respiratory physiology, particularly the control of breathing. To get him to teach me about uptake and distribution, I (and fate) would have to supply the stimulus. John was the brilliant sparkler, shedding light everywhere. But for John, his nitrous oxide experiment was a wonderful one-off. He had moved on. Fortunately, something beyond his control brought John back to uptake and distribution. I was in the right place at the right time (**Figure 6.1**). More about that in a moment.

Being John's fellow was like living in a grownup version of the Hyde Park School for Little Children. Every Monday morning John held the fellow's meeting. *Show and Tell!* Admission to the Bookhouse! I learned what everyone was doing and told the group what I'd done the previous week and would do the next week. I loved it. As I grew academically, my love of it increased. I pushed John to continue his fellow's meetings long after the time he felt they were no longer necessary. Later, when I had fellows, I held my own Monday Lab Meeting.

By the late 1960s, I went my own way in the world of research, focusing on quantitating the effects of inhaled anesthetics and defining the factors that governed inhaled anesthetic pharmacokinetics. I went on to explore the mechanisms by which inhaled anesthetics act. My formal fellowship with John ended.

Nevertheless, in my mind, I was, and always remained, a Severinghaus fellow.

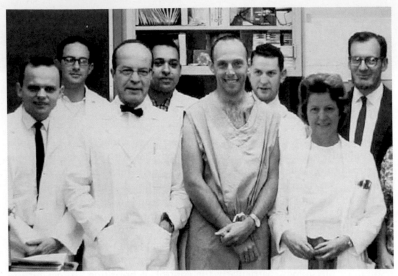

Figure 6.1 University of California, San Francisco research team. (Left to right): Cedric Bainton, Larry Saidman, Bob Mitchell, A. Freeman Bradley, Ted Eger, Ed Munson, Dorothy Herbert, and John Severinghaus.

How Fast Does CO$_2$ Increase in an Apneic Patient?

When I'd settled in, John gave me the first of several assignments in respiratory physiology research: measure the rate at which arterial PCO$_2$ (PaCO$_2$) increases when a patient stops breathing (apnea), an increase that stimulates breathing and thus determines how quickly a patient might breathe after anesthesia.[3] In part, the change simply reflects the rate at which the body makes CO$_2$. It also reflects the body's capacity to store the CO$_2$ that it makes. That is, it reflects the solubility and buffering of CO$_2$ in tissues. *Aha! An uptake problem!* Being in John's lab, I knew that the end-tidal PCO$_2$ (PACO$_2$) approximately equaled the arterial PCO$_2$ (PaCO$_2$). So, I just had to measure the end-tidal CO$_2$ in an apneic subject. This seemed like a contradiction, *how can an apneic patient have an end-tidal anything?* We approximated that by having patients rebreathe from a small (400 mL) bag loaded with air containing their initial CO$_2$ concentration,[3] finding that CO$_2$ in the small bag increased at a steady-state rate of 2 to 4 mm Hg/min. It increased faster in the first minute as the lungs went from equilibrating with the arterial CO$_2$ to equilibrating with the greater CO$_2$ in venous blood, perhaps 8 to 10 mm Hg greater. Hypothermia slowed the rate of rise, partly because metabolism decreased and partly because the solubility of CO$_2$ increased.

High-altitude Physiology

John supported my fascination with inhaled anesthetic kinetics and dynamics but never pursued them as I did. He took me and other fellows to work in the high-altitude laboratory on White Mountain at 12,000 ft. I remember falling asleep in the communal dormitory, listening to the breathing around me, breathing stimulated by the diminished oxygen partial pressure at high altitude. One individual exhibited a particularly interesting breathing pattern, a Cheyne-Stokes pattern in which his breathing increased and then faded away and stopped. I suddenly awoke from my reverie, terrified at the realization that I had stopped breathing.

John took a sabbatical in 1966 just as I was finishing the research on carbon dioxide pharmacology. Fearing I would be at loose ends, John set me a task with the ever-delightful Ralph Kellogg and others, including Allan Mines. We tested the thesis that a sustained (8-hour) decrease in $PACO_2$ would shift the resting $PACO_2$ versus ventilation curve to the left and that the shift would be larger if hypoxia accompanied the sustained decrease. As our report noted,[4] during the 8-hour period of acclimatization, the subject *"was allowed to read, watch television (I Love Lucy was a favorite), or do nothing; at no time was he allowed to sleep."* We did many things to keep each subject awake, the most effective being a blast of air in his ear. The experiment included studies of the effect of administering several combinations of oxygen and carbon dioxide for 8 hours (only one combination for a given 8-hour period). The combination of decreased oxygen and increased carbon dioxide was particularly unpleasant. The resulting stimulation of breathing and a sense of claustrophobia kept subjects awake without the blast of air in the ear. *I couldn't deal with the claustrophobia and declined to be a subject!* The results confirmed the above thesis.

The Incidental Invention of MAC

In the second year of my fellowship, John handed Giles Merkel (another fellow) and me a bottle containing a clear fluid, halopropane, a new anesthetic made by Dow Chemical Co. *"Would we like to define its properties?"* John asked. *"Of course,"* we replied. *"But how do we do that?"* We were told to figure it out. Defining the properties might be as simple as determining the effect of an anesthetizing concentration of halopropane on vital functions such as respiration or circulation. By now I was a member of the Cardiovascular Research Institute, so that shouldn't be a problem after we divined what anesthetizing concentration to use.

But the problem was greater than that. One really wanted to know whether halopropane was better, worse, or just different from the other clinical anesthetics of the day, particularly halothane. That meant that we needed a standard of anesthetic potency that would allow us to determine the properties of halopropane and halothane at concentrations of identical anesthetic effect (ie, equipotent concentrations)—and multiples of that concentration. Only then would we be comparing apples to apples. But there was no standard. We would have to invent one. How we would measure the concentration was preordained in John's lab. We would measure the end-tidal (alveolar) anesthetic concentration (F_A) because that immediately reflected the arterial anesthetic partial pressure, just as it might for CO_2. If maintained for sufficient time, F_A would also reflect the anesthetic partial pressure in the central nervous system, the site where the anesthetic acted.

What anesthetic effect would a clinical anesthetist agree was a hallmark of anesthesia? It would have to be something that all inhaled anesthetics caused. That excluded many anesthetic side effects, even clinically important side effects such as nausea and vomiting, blood pressure changes, or muscle relaxation. Some anesthetics produced little nausea and vomiting; some a lot. The anesthetic effect couldn't be blood pressure changes: cyclopropane increased blood pressure; halothane caused a decrease. It couldn't be relaxation: halothane produced muscle relaxation; nitrous oxide caused rigidity. Although eye signs such as pupillary dilation might be clinically useful for a specific anesthetic, they varied from anesthetic to anesthetic. Unusable endpoints! But all inhaled anesthetics caused one clinically useful endpoint: immobility in the face of a noxious stimulus (eg, a surgical incision). Surgeons became grumpy if their patient moved during surgery.

At Monday morning show and tell, we discussed that we could compare inhaled anesthetics by determining the minimum alveolar concentration—the F_A—required to produce immobility in 50% of subjects receiving a supramaximal noxious stimulus such as skin incision. In dogs an electrical stimulus or pinching the tail could provide the noxious stimulus. John invented the acronym, MAC, noting the parallel to the acronym describing the speed of sound. Lighthearted and serious comments accompanied the name.

Now Giles and I could compare halothane and halopropane and determine whether one was better, worse, or just different.[5] Larry Saidman had joined the group and determined the effect of morphine premedication and the addition of nitrous oxide on the MAC of halothane in patients. He used that surgical incision as the supramaximal noxious stimulus, and first presented his findings at the New York Postgraduate Assembly.[6] I'm told he was nervous, and became more nervous when one of the grand old men of anesthesia, Louis Orkin, rose to comment. In his booming, gloriously nasal New York accent, Orkin said that MAC wasn't new. Larry felt faint. *"Yes,"* Orkin continued, *"We've always known about MAC. When the surgeon makes an incision and the patient moves, the surgeon says 'Hey, MAC!'"*

Thus, was born MAC, the minimum alveolar concentration—the F_A—required to produce immobility in 50% of subjects receiving a supramaximal noxious

Minimum Alveolar Anesthetic Concentration: A Standard of Anesthetic Potency

Edmond I. Eger, II, M.D.,* Lawrence J. Saiman, M.D.,†
Bernard Brandstater, M.B., F.F.A.R.C.S.‡

The minimum alveolar concentration of anesthetic (MAC) necessary to prevent movement in response to a painful stimulus was relatively constant in dogs anesthettized with halothane. MAC varied over a two-fold range with the intensity of the stimulus, but appeared to reach an upper limit beyond which a further increase in intensity did not increase MAC. For the same stimulus MAC was constant from dog to dog. MAC was unaffected by duration of anesthesia, unaltered by hypocarbia or hypercarbia. by phenylephrine.induced hypertension or by mild hypoxia (Pao_2, 30 to 60 mm. of mercury). Hemorrhagic hypoten. sion or marked acute metabolic acidosis reduced MAC by 10 to 20 per cent. Severe hypoxia (Pao_2 less than 30 mm. of mercury) reduced MAC by 25 to 50 per cent.

MAC appears to be a useful standard by which all inhalation anethetics may be compared.

In 1963 Merkel and Eger described a technique for the determination in dogs of the minimum alveolar concentration of anesthetic (MAC) required to prevent gross muscular movement in response to a painful stimulus.[1] The alveolar concentration •• was chosen as

* Assistant Clinical Professor, Department of Anesthesia, and Associate Staff Member, Cardiovascular Research Institute, University of California Medical Center, San Francisco, California.
† Research Trainee. Department of Anesthesia, University of California Medical Center, San Francisco,California.
‡ Chariman, Department of Anesthesia, American University of Beirut. Beirut, Lebanon.
Accepted for publication July 7, 1965. Sup ported in part by United States Public Health Service Grants 5-K3-GM-17,685; 5RO1 HE07946; 5Tl GM-63; and HE06285.
•• In this and the succeeding papers concerning MAC, we will use alveolar concentration (volumes per cent) rather than partial pressure. However, concentration will always be described relative to a pressure of one atmosphere (760 mm. of mercury). For those who would prefer partial pressure, our figures may be converted to atmospheres pressure simply by moving the decimal point two places to the left .

the most readily measured index of brain anesthetic tension. The dogs were anesthetized with a small dose of thiopental and anesthesia was maintained thereafter with either halothane or halopropane. The concentration required to produce unresponsiveness was found to be fairly constant in al one dog regardless of duration of anesthesia. This apparent reproducibility led us to believe that MAC might be useful as a standard of anesthetic potency. Potency may be defined as the reciprocal of MAC, or potency equals 1/MAC. Thus, nitrous oxide would be less potent than cyclopropane, and cyclopropane less potent than halothane. A standard such as MAC would allow a comparison of respiratory or circulatory (or other) effects produced by equipotent doses of two or more anesthetics. However, before general use for this purpose, we must know the limits of reproducibility of MAC and whether it is affected by such things as intensity of the painful stimulus, duration of anesthesia, hypocarbia, hypercarbia, hypotension, hypertension, hypoxia, or metabolic acidosis. We have attempted to answer the above questions in this study.

Methods and Results

The technique previously described was altered slightly in that thiopental was not used. Anesthesia was induced and maintained with oxygen plus the gas to he studied (usually halothane). This change was made after discovery that an induction dose of thiopental (150 to 200 mg.) reduced MAC by 5 to 20 per cent for 2 to 4 hours . Rusy *et al.,*[2] similarly found that the anesthetic effect of 225 mg. of thiopental on cyclopropane requirement in dogs was apparent 45 minutes or longer after injection. At least in dogs. thiopental may have a more than evanescent

Figure 6.2 Paper suggesting that the concentration of anesthetic associated with loss of response to noxious stimulation be adopted as a standard measure of potency. (From Eger Elll, Saidman LJ, Brandstater B. Minimum alveolar anesthetic concentration: a standard of anesthetic potency. *Anesthesiology.* 1965;26:756-763.)

stimulus. We published a paper suggesting that this be adopted as a standard measure of the potency of inhaled anesthetics (**Figure 6.2**).[5,7] It has been the standard ever since.

Some anesthetists suggested that MAC should be MAP because pressure and not concentration determines immobility. That is, the capacity of anesthetic molecules at the anesthetic site of action to produce immobility must reflect the number of molecules at the site, and the number is proportional to the partial pressure in blood and not to concentration in blood or the alveoli. The fraction of alveolar gas (F_A) that produces immobility at sea level would be less than the F_A at Leadville, Colorado, at 10,000 ft elevation, but the partial pressure would be the same.

This comment was correct, but too late. The name MAC had been established, had been connected with the concept, and it seemed to flow off the tongue (or, at least, off of my tongue). So, we patched the definition instead of changing the name. MAC became the minimum alveolar concentration *at sea level* that produced immobility in 50% of patients subjected to a supramaximal noxious stimulus. The "at sea level" converted the concentration to a partial pressure.

MAC in Various Flavors

Refinements followed. MAC provided but one point: the concentration on a dose-response curve at which immobility was obtained. Half MAC was not the point at which half immobility was obtained. Half of a MAC had no meaning other than being the concentration that was half that producing immobility. Other responses on the dose-response curve for this magical thing called anesthesia were developed, responses often analogous to MAC in the manner of their determination but different in their meaning. Thus, in 1970, Stoelting gave us MAC-awake, the alveolar concentration suppressing appropriate responses to commands such as "Open your eyes" or "Squeeze my hand" in 50% of subjects.[8] Roizen gave us MAC-BAR, the alveolar concentration suppressing autonomic reflex responses (eg, increase in blood pressure or heart rate) to noxious stimulation.[9]

What Might Be Done With MAC?

The potential uses of MAC, itself, became clear. MAC defined the F_A needed for clinical anesthesia. It provided a yardstick for anesthetic comparisons. It allowed the quantitative definition of factors that altered anesthetic potency, factors such as aging or body temperature. It would be used to test theories of narcosis.

Not everyone viewed these possibilities as opportunities. My father asked me what I was doing. When I outlined my dreams (eg, pinching the tails of dogs), he questioned whether I was pursuing a career as a real doctor. He wasn't alone. Soon after we published the first paper on MAC, Dr. Cullen called me into his office and asked what I was going to do next. I didn't know what to say; we had just invented something that provided a lifetime's work. Giles Merkel and I talked about the doors that MAC opened for studies of comparative pharmacology, studies that would change anesthesia. We had a world of opportunities we might share, but Giles had become a fellow as a 1-year lark and that was done. He would go into private practice, and I was left to do as I pleased with MAC.

That gave me worlds that some dear people thought offered dubious opportunities. Nonetheless, these opportunities would govern much of my life for a half-century. For the next 2 decades, I worked with numerous colleagues to develop many of the major concepts in pharmacokinetics. Over the same time plus two more decades, I would define the comparative pharmacology of inhaled anesthetics. And these studies prompted other research studies, explorations of how inhaled anesthetics affected the mind and whether new and better inhaled anesthetics could be found. The search for new and better anesthetics and how these might affect the mind led to investigations in the 1990s of theories of narcosis. I would pursue these studies with young and old fellows and faculty as part of a radical change in the world of anesthesia, a change from a qualitative to a quantitative understanding of what we anesthetists did in the delivery of anesthesia. We facilitated a change in anesthesia from an art to a science.

These worlds were connected. My first and true love, my addiction, my mistress, was pharmacokinetics (what the body did to the anesthetics), this geometry of anatomy, physiology, and physics that made pictures in my head. Pictures, always pictures. Comparative pharmacology added pharmacodynamics (what anesthetics do to the body) to pharmacokinetics. Anesthetics affected their kinetics by how they altered breathing and the output of the heart. Anesthetics altered the distribution of ventilation and the distribution of blood flow, and these, too, altered kinetics.

References

1. Severinghaus JW. The rate of uptake of nitrous oxide in man. *J Clin Invest.* 1954;33:1183-1189.
2. Severinghaus JW, Larson CP, Eger EI. Correction factors for infrared carbon dioxide pressure broadening by nitrogen, nitrous oxide and cyclopropane. *Anesthesiology.* 1961;22:429-432.
3. Eger EI, Severinghaus JW. The rate of rise of $PaCO_2$ in the apneic anesthetized patient. *Anesthesiology.* 1961;22:419-425.

4. Eger EI II, Kellogg RH, Mines AH, Lima-Ostos M, Morrill CG, Kent DW. Influence of CO_2 on ventilatory acclimatization to altitude. *J Appl Physiol.* 1968;24:607-615.

5. Merkel G, Eger EI II. A comparative study of halothane and halopropane anesthesia including method for determining equipotency. *Anesthesiology.* 1963;24:346-357.

6. Saidman LJ, Eger EI II. Effect of nitrous oxide and of narcotic premedication on the alveolar concentration of halothane required for anesthesia. *Anesthesiology.* 1964;25:302-306.

7. Eger EI II, Saidman LJ, Brandstater B. Minimum alveolar anesthetic concentration: a standard of anesthetic potency. *Anesthesiology.* 1965;26:756-763.

8. Stoelting RK, Longnecker DE, Eger EI II. Minimal alveolar concentrations on awakening from methoxyflurane, halothane, ether and fluroxene in man: MAC awake. *Anesthesiology.* 1970;33:5-9.

9. Roizen MF, Horrigan RW, Frazer BM. Anesthetic doses blocking adrenergic (stress) and cardiovascular responses to incision—MAC BAR. *Anesthesiology.* 1981;54:390-398.

The Evolution of MAC

7

Toward a Better Definition of MAC

As described in Chapter 6, Giles Merkel and I collaborated from 1961 through 1963[1] to define the anesthetic potency of halopropane in dogs. For our measure of potency, we settled on the minimum alveolar concentration (MAC) of halopropane that rendered 50% of the dogs unresponsive to tail clamping or electrical stimulation (they proved to be equivalently unpleasant). A year later, Larry Saidman and I extended the concept to humans (**Figure 7.1**).[2] We used reaction to surgical incision as the noxious stimulus, since response to electric current wasn't particularly interesting in humans and tail clamping wasn't an option. Our results showed that the addition of morphine premedication slightly decreased MAC for halothane, whereas concurrently administering nitrous oxide caused a dramatic reduction of MAC for halothane.

Larry and I enlisted the assistance of Bernard Brandstater, with whom I had previously collaborated to determine the solubility of methoxyflurane in rubber.[3] This was useful because rubber was used in anesthesia circuits, altering anesthetic uptake. Additionally, primitive "anesthesia meters" were based on anesthetics taking the stretch out of rubber bands, with the result appearing on a calibrated scale.

In 1965, Brandstater, Saidman and I published three reports that refined the concept of MAC.[4-6] The first of these showed that MAC as defined by the use of a supramaximal stimulus was constant from dog to dog (**Table 7.1**).[4] We further showed that perturbations that did not unduly stress the central nervous system did not alter MAC. For example, increasing duration of anesthesia did not change MAC. Similarly, modest hypocapnia or hypercapnia did not affect MAC. Neither phenylephrine-induced hypertension, nor mild hypoxia (Pao_2 of 30-60 mm Hg) significantly changed MAC. We found that MAC decreased in certain potentially life-threatening situations. For example, severe hypoxia (Pao_2 <30 mm Hg) decreased MAC 25% to 50%. Hemorrhagic hypotension or marked metabolic acidosis might decrease MAC by 10% to 20%. We also noted that it was the absolute partial pressure that determined anesthetic effect, not the fraction of inspired gas. Therefore, we recommended that MAC, expressed as a percent of inspired gas, should always be calculated to reflect a partial pressure at sea level.

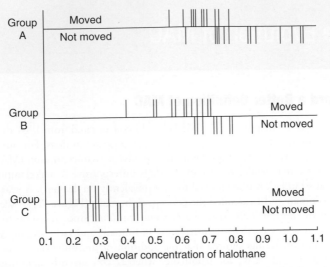

Figure 7.1 Alveolar concentrations associated with moving/not moving, for halothane (group A), halothane with morphine premedication (group B), and halothane with nitrous oxide (group C). (From Saidman LJ, Eger El II. Effect of nitrous oxide and of narcotic premedication on the alveolar concentration of halothane required for anesthesia. *Anesthesiology*. 1964;25:302-306.)

Our next report found that the MAC values of halothane and cyclopropane correlated directly with changes in body temperature.[5] The correlation of MAC and temperature has clinical implications and also provides insight into possible mechanisms of inhaled anesthetic action. The correlation was steeper with the more potent, more lipid-soluble halothane.

We then reported MAC values for clinically and experimentally available volatile anesthetics: methoxyflurane, halothane, diethyl ether, fluroxene, cyclopropane, xenon, and nitrous oxide in dogs (**Figure 7.2**).[6] This report provided the first of several forays into mechanisms of action by noting the correlation of MAC values with lipophilicity of the anesthetic examined, a finding consistent with the "theory" (really an observed correlation) proposed earlier by Meyer[7] and Overton (**Figure 7.3**).[8]

MAC Matures

The concept of MAC became fundamental to understanding inhaled anesthetic pharmacology. MAC became our primary research tool for describing the essence of anesthesia itself.

Table 7.1 MAC for Halothane in Dogs, Documenting That It Is Highly Stable

Stimulus	Dog 1	Dog 2	Dog 3	Mean
Tail clamp	0.89	0.85	0.68	0.81
Tail clamp, plus end- tidal CO_2 of 57 mm Hg	0.93	0.89	0.60	0.80
10 V	0.80	0.70	0.47	0.66
30 V	0.98	0.82	0.68	0.83
50 V	0.98	0.82	0.71	0.84
Endotracheal tube	0.89	0.52	0.35	0.55
Incision	0.80	0.52	0.79	0.69
Paw clamp	0.50	0.64	0.35	0.50
Spontaneous movement	0.50	0.52	0.35	0.46

From Eger EIII, Saidman LJ, Brandstater B. Minimum alveolar anesthetic concentration: a standard of anesthetic potency. *Anesthesiology*. 1965;26:756-763.

We studied the relationship between MAC and other vital aspects of anesthesia (eg, MAC_{awake},[9] the end-tidal anesthetic concentration that prevents voluntary responses to spoken commends in 50% of subjects). We used MAC to explore the anesthetic effects of extremes of physiological challenge. For example, MAC does not bear a constant relationship to the anesthetic concentration required to produce apnea, a finding suggesting that the margin of safety differs among anesthetics.[10] The decrease in MAC associated with a decrease in body temperature varied among anesthetics, being greater with more lipid soluble anesthetics.[5,10] As noted above, modest changes in the partial pressure of carbon dioxide, PCO_2, had little effect on MAC in dogs, but greater changes decreased MAC, causing anesthesia from CO_2 at a bit more than a third of an atmosphere of CO_2.[11] Drugs that decreased central nervous system concentrations of norepinephrine decreased MAC, and conversely a drug that increased those concentrations increased MAC.[12]

Age affects MAC. In 1969, George Gregory published his classic study of the effect of age on halothane MAC in children and adults (**Figure 7.4**), showing that MAC progressively decreased from a high in the first few months of life except, perhaps, for a small upward bump at adolescence.[13]

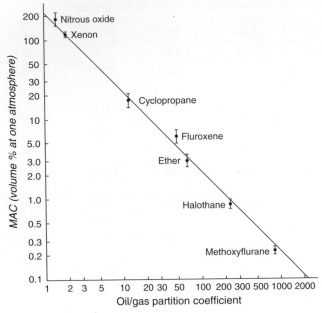

Figure 7.2 The high correlation between lipid solubility and anesthetic potency based on minimum alveolar concentration (MAC). (From Eger El II, Brandstater B, Saidman LJ, Regan MJ, Severinghaus JW, Munson ES. Equipotent alveolar concentrations of methoxyflurane, halothane, diethyl ether, fluroxene, cyclopropane, xenon and nitrous oxide in the dog. *Anesthesiology*. 1965;26:771-777.)

Six years after Gregory published his work, Wendell Stevens performed the same study using isoflurane as the anesthetic, finding parallel effects of aging in adults.[14] Unfortunately, *Anesthesiology* initially rejected Steven's study because the editors believed there were too many "me too" studies using MAC. *Those damn editors!* Stevens persisted, and the editors relented. Steven's paper is one of the hundred most cited papers in the field of anesthesia.

The interchange with *Anesthesiology* changed my thoughts on submissions and journals. Until the time of Stevens' submission of the isoflurane MAC paper, I had routinely sent my work to *Anesthesiology*, the most prestigious journal in the specialty. Stevens' interchange with the editors of *Anesthesiology* made it clear that our specialty needed two prestigious journals to spur competition. Thereafter I sent my work to *Anesthesia and Analgesia* and urged other investigators to do likewise. Not many listened, but I liked being Don Quixote.

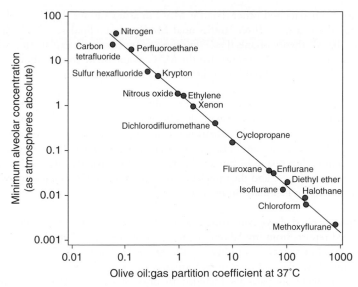

Figure 7.3 The correlation between lipid solubility (olive oil:gas partition coefficient) and anesthetic potency based on minimum alveolar concentration (MAC). (Data from Meyer HH. Theorie der Alkoholnarkose. *Arch Exptl Pathol Pharmakol.* 1899;42:109-118 and Overton E. *Studien über die Narkose, Zugleich ein Beitrag zur allgemeinen Pharmakologie.* Gustav Fischer; 1901:1-195.)

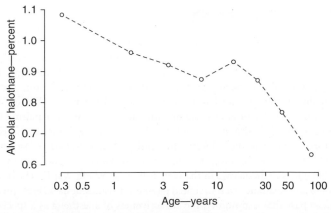

Figure 7.4 The decrease in minimum alveolar concentration (MAC) with increasing age. (From Gregory GA, Eger EI II, Munson ES. The relationship between age and halothane requirement in man. *Anesthesiology.* 1969;30:488-491.)

We used our data and other data for MAC to assess various theories explaining anesthetic action. Three studies used MAC to test a lipid versus a hydrate (water-based) theory of anesthesia, finding a more consistent explanation with the lipid theory.[15-17] We found that the MAC of anesthetic combinations were additive,[18,19] as they should be if they act by a common mechanism.[20]

MAC became a unifying measurement to calibrate the effects of anesthetic dose on vital functions and to compare the effects of different anesthetics on such functions. MAC facilitated comparison of the respiratory effects of ether versus methoxyflurane in humans[21]; the cardiovascular effects of halothane, fluroxene, ether, and cyclopropane in humans[22]; the epileptic capacities of nine inhaled anesthetics in dogs[23]; and the interaction of neuromuscular blocking drugs with isoflurane versus halothane in patients.[24]

The papers cited above constitute a small sample of the more than 500 peer-reviewed reports from my laboratory, most focused on anesthetic kinetics and dynamics. In one way or another, most of my research leveraged MAC and the concepts of uptake and distribution kinetics I had developed. In more recent years, my focus increasingly included theories of narcosis. However, MAC proved fundamental in understanding mechanisms of anesthesia. We defined anesthesia as immobility in response to noxious stimulation, based on the concept of MAC. We therefore rejected as mechanisms of anesthetic action any proposal that could not explain immobility.

A Change in the Specialty

Anesthesiology came into its own as a premiere specialty in the 20th century. Many factors led to its mid-century rise. The foundation for our specialty had been set by John Snow (a founder of both anesthesia and epidemiology). Ralph Waters envisioned anesthesiology as an academic discipline, planting the seeds for virtually all modern academic anesthesiology departments. World War II advanced the practice of anesthesia by bifurcating the tasks of repairing injury to the surgeon while the anesthesiologist kept the patient alive. To meet the needs for military anesthesiologists, the United States drafted physicians and trained them as anesthesiologists. This vastly increased the pool of physicians specializing in anesthesia care in the years following World War II. The development of health insurance that included payment for anesthesia services provided a financial base that maintained the attractiveness of anesthesia as a specialty.

Lastly, the production of the atomic bomb led, indirectly, to the synthesis of halothane, the first fluorinated inhaled anesthetic. Gas centrifugation is one of the more effective mechanisms for separating fissile ^{235}U from stable ^{238}U. In this process, uranium is combined with fluorine to produce uranium hexafluoride, UF_6. The fluorine chemistry to create UF_6 was developed by Imperial Chemical Industries (ICI) during World War II. After the war, ICI turned to developing pharmaceuticals. Their expertise with fluorine enabled synthesis of novel fluorinated hydrocarbon anesthetics. The first of these to be commercially successful was halothane, whose physical properties and chemical stability led to all modern fluorinated inhaled anesthetics, including isoflurane, desflurane, and sevoflurane, today the most widely used inhaled anesthetics in the world.

Perspective

My UCSF colleagues and I created MAC to enable our own research. However, we expected our definition of MAC to be broadly useful in anesthesia research, allowing investigators to describe anesthetic potency and pharmacological effects in consistent terms that were clinically relevant: as fractions of the steady-state partial pressure at sea level that prevented movement. We also thought that by using a clinically meaningful definition, lack of movement during surgery, clinicians might find the concept useful. Reality exceeded our optimistic expectations.

I believe our development of MAC, and our mathematically precise descriptions of uptake and distribution, played a major role in the rise of anesthesia as a premiere specialty. MAC and understanding uptake and distribution transformed the administration of anesthesia from an art to a science. MAC for inhaled anesthetics enabled and encouraged quantification of anesthetic effects on the body as well as what the body did to anesthetics. Attempts have been made to replicate the concepts of MAC for intravenous drugs, but these lack the elegance of MAC because alveolar concentrations can be observed in real time, while intravenous drug concentrations are only known after the fact. MAC and an appreciation of the inhaled anesthetic kinetics prompted universal application of end-tidal anesthetic analysis. A vast body of information now exists on the physiological consequences of anesthetics, consequences revealed by studies applying MAC. Many young physicians are drawn to our specialty because of our ability to measure our interventions with such precision and immediacy.

I am proud to have been part of this journey of discovery. Although I went into anesthesia for money and power, my pride in discovery has been a greater reward.

Did I invent MAC, under the guidance of John Severinghaus, and with considerable assistance from Merkel, Saidman, Brandstater, and others? Or is MAC merely a property of specific molecules, and of the biology that mediates anesthetic action. The property exists in nature. Perhaps my colleagues and I merely observed and reported this property as we traveled along our research journeys, just as Meyer and Overton observed the correlation between anesthetic potency and lipophilicity decades earlier.

It doesn't matter. As Richard Feynman said "*the prize is the pleasure of finding the thing out, the kick in the discovery, the observation that other people use it. Those are the real things.*"[25]

References

1. Merkel G, Eger EI II. A comparative study of halothane and halopropane anesthesia including method for determining equipotency. *Anesthesiology*. 1963;24:346-357.
2. Saidman LJ, Eger EI II. Effect of nitrous oxide and of narcotic premedication on the alveolar concentration of halothane required for anesthesia. *Anesthesiology*. 1964;25:302-306.
3. Eger EI II, Brandstater B. Solubility of methoxyflurane in rubber. *Anesthesiology*. 1963;24:679-683.
4. Eger EI II, Saidman LJ, Brandstater B. Minimum alveolar anesthetic concentration: a standard of anesthetic potency. *Anesthesiology*. 1965;26:756-763.
5. Eger EI II, Saidman LJ, Brandstater B. Temperature dependence of halothane and cyclopropane anesthesia in dogs: correlation with some theories of anesthetic action. *Anesthesiology*. 1965;26:764-770.
6. Eger EI II, Brandstater B, Saidman LJ, Regan MJ, Severinghaus JW, Munson ES. Equipotent alveolar concentrations of methoxyflurane, halothane, diethyl ether, fluroxene, cyclopropane, xenon and nitrous oxide in the dog. *Anesthesiology*. 1965;26:771-777.
7. Meyer HH. Theorie der Alkoholnarkose. *Arch Exptl Pathol Pharmakol*. 1899;42:109-118.
8. Overton E. *Studien über die Narkose, Zugleich ein Beitrag zur allgemeinen Pharmakologie*. Gustav Fischer; 1901:1-195.
9. Stoelting RK, Longnecker DE, Eger EI II. Minimal alveolar concentrations on awakening from methoxyflurane, halothane, ether and fluroxene in man: MAC awake. *Anesthesiology*. 1970;33:5-9.
10. Regan MJ, Eger EI II. Effect of hypothermia in dogs on anesthetizing and apneic doses of inhalation agents. Determination of the anesthetic index (Apnea/MAC). *Anesthesiology*. 1967;28:689-700.
11. Eisele JH, Eger EI II, Muallem M. Narcotic properties of carbon dioxide in the dog. *Anesthesiology*. 1967;28:856-865.
12. Miller RD, Way WL, Eger EI II. The effects of alpha-methyldopa, reserpine, guanethidine, and iproniazid on minimum alveolar anesthetic requirement (MAC). *Anesthesiology*. 1968;29:1153-1158.
13. Gregory GA, Eger EI II, Munson ES. The relationship between age and halothane requirement in man. *Anesthesiology*. 1969;30:488-491.

14. Stevens WC, Dolan WM, Gibbons RT, et al. Minimum alveolar concentrations (MAC) of isoflurane with and without nitrous oxide in patients of various ages. *Anesthesiology*. 1975;42:197-200.

15. Eger EI II, Lundgren C, Miller SL, Stevens WC. Anesthetic potencies of sulfur hexafluoride, carbon tetrafluoride, chloroform and Ethrane in dogs: correlation with the hydrate and lipid theories of anesthetic action. *Anesthesiology*. 1969;30:129-135.

16. Eger EI II, Shargel RO. The lack of hydrate formation at a temperature of 0 C of methoxyflurane, halothane, diethyl ether and fluroxene. *Anesthesiology*. 1969;30:136-137.

17. Miller SL, Eger EI II, Lundgren C. Anaesthetic potency of CF4 and SF6 in dogs. *Nature*. 1969;221:468-469.

18. Miller RD, Wahrenbrock EA, Schroeder CF, Knipstein TW, Eger EI II, Buechel DR. Ethylene-halothane anesthesia: addition or synergism? *Anesthesiology*. 1969;31:301-304.

19. Cullen SC, Eger EI II, Cullen BF, Gregory P. Observations on the anesthetic effect of the combination of xenon and halothane. *Anesthesiology*. 1969;31:305-309.

20. Shafer SL, Hendrickx JF, Flood P, Sonner J, Eger EI II. Additivity versus synergy: a theoretical analysis of implications for anesthetic mechanisms. *Anesth Analg*. 2008;107:507-524.

21. Larson CP Jr, Eger EI II, Muallem M, Buechel DR, Munson ES, Eisele JH. The effects of diethyl ether and methoxyflurane on ventilation: II. A comparative study in man. *Anesthesiology*. 1969;30:174-184.

22. Eger EI II, Smith NT, Cullen DJ, Cullen BF, Gregory GA. A comparison of the cardiovascular effects of halothane, fluroxene, ether and cyclopropane in man: a resume. *Anesthesiology*. 1971;34:25-41.

23. Joas TA, Stevens WC, Eger EI II. Electroencephalographic seizure activity in dogs during anaesthesia. *Br J Anaesth*. 1971;43:739-745.

24. Miller RD, Eger EI II, Way WL, Stevens WC, Dolan WM. Comparative neuromuscular effects of Forane and halothane alone and in combination with d-tubocurarine in man. *Anesthesiology*. 1971;35:38-42.

25. Feynman R. *The Pleasure of Finding Things Out*. BBC Interview; 1981. Accessed April 1, 2019. https://videos.cern.ch/record/1055846

The Evolution of Pharmacokinetics

8

Continuing Studies of Uptake

To understand the action of anesthetic drugs, I needed to understand the process by which the drugs enter the body and are transported to the brain and other tissues. These are basic principles of physics (eg, flow and diffusion), chemistry (eg, solubility), and physiology (eg, metabolism). In my days on the third floor of the Fort Leavenworth hospital, I expressed these concepts in equations. My differential equations provided precise, testable descriptions of the processes of anesthetic uptake and distribution.

John was not particularly interested in my studies of uptake and distribution when I became his fellow. However, he saw that this was important to me and accepted my initiatives. To pursue my mathematical models required resources beyond clinical laboratories. Fortunately, the University of California at San Francisco was a world-class medical school with all the trimmings. I took a course in Fortran and worked with the teacher to express my equations in that language. One cool spring night we converted our Fortran code into punch cards and read those into Berkeley's massive IBM computer. Who could not be impressed by a computer with so many vacuum tubes that it required an air conditioned building just to keep from melting. We pressed the GO button and awaited the result. Streams of neatly folded pages, each with hundreds of lines of results flowed out of the printer. Within a few minutes on that cool spring Berkeley night my equations produced a year's worth of Ft. Leavenworth work. I now had predictions that I could experimentally test.

In John's lab, I'd learned to use the infrared analyzer to measure CO_2. John had other infrared analyzers that measured nearly all inhaled anesthetics, and I learned to use those, too. We pushed these analyzers to their limit to determine anesthetic solubilities in blood, tissues, and the materials in the anesthetic circuits used to deliver anesthetics to patients.[1] However, as our research progressed, we needed ever greater sensitivity in our assays. We learned about something called a gas chromatograph, a device that increased our reach a million-fold. We purchased one, and then two.

The Meeting on Uptake and Distribution in New York

In 1961, a wonderful event brought John back to uptake and distribution. In that year, Emanuel Papper, the chairman of the Department of Anesthesiology at Columbia University, invited John to participate in a 1962 Conference on Anesthetic Uptake and Distribution (the first conference on the topic). As a good mentor, John saw to it that I was also invited to participate. All my efforts, equations, predictions, and ideas would have a forum!

In 1960, Henry Price used principles of blood flow and tissue solubility to explain the distribution of thiopental after intravenous injection.[2] This work led John,[3] Thomas MacKrell,[4] and William Mapleson[5] to predict the uptake and distribution of inhaled anesthetics using the same concepts. I also incorporated Price's work into my equations. However, John, Thomas, and William used mathematical approximations (rather than my exact iterative approach) to predict the uptake and distribution of inhaled anesthetics. They applied their equations to the rates of increase of the alveolar (F_A) to inspired (F_I) anesthetic concentrations (the F_A/F_I ratio), which they presented at the conference. However, I knew that their approximations were incorrect because they did not predict the effect of the inspired concentration, the concentration effect.

At the meeting John and Tom MacKrell spoke first, presenting the predictions of uptake and distribution from their work with simulation models based on resisters and capacitors. I went next, presenting the results of my differential equations solved computationally at Berkeley. I showed that the approximate equations used by John and Tom could not correctly incorporate dynamic aspects such as the nonlinear influence of inspired concentration of a gas on its own rate of uptake. William Mapleson presented his results last. This wry Welshman started by saying his "...talk was in shambles." He thought he offered novel solutions, but Severinghaus and MacKrell had already presented nearly identical work. Even worse, I showed that their work was incomplete, as it could not predict either the concentration or the second gas effects.

As is so often the case, their work was not "wrong," per se, but simply incomplete. Science advances from initial approximations of the truth to better approximations. My differential equations were a better mathematical model than their simulations based on resisters and capacitors. As expected, yet better models came along. For example, none of us had paid attention to the work of William Perl, who rightly pointed out in 1960 that uptake might be influenced by the movement of gas from one tissue to an adjacent tissue, eg, intertissue diffusion.[6] He repeated this possibility at the conference.[7] Of course, he was right, and our models evolved to accommodate more data.

The proceedings of the 1962 New York conference were published the following year. For the anesthesia community, this led to a seminal transformation by quantifying the movement of anesthetics into and throughout the body. It was a major contribution to the evolution of anesthesia from a clinical art into a quantitative science. It was the culmination of my thoughts that began with my 1958 conversation with John after his lecture to Iowa residents. I had filled my days at Fort Leavenworth with differential equations that yielded their predictions only through laborious calculation. These calculations predicted the effect of differential blood flow and solubility on anesthetic distribution, and underlay the fortuitous discovery of the concentration effect.[8] The conference participants shared the conclusions that differential tissue blood flow as well as solubility determined the effect site concentrations of anesthetics.

My work prompted Dr. Cullen to invite me to apply for an NIH Research Career Development Award, something that would provide financial support for full-time research. John would mentor me for five more years. "Yes!" I said, addicted to what I was doing and might do with John. And so my 1- or 2-year sojourn in California extended to forever. What follows is more of a scientific odyssey than a personal autobiography, a journey that largely took place starting in the 1960s and continuing through the 1970s, and beyond.

Solubility Was the Key

My earliest work, the construction of the differential equations describing the travel of anesthetics into and throughout the body, relied on solubility values determined by other investigators. But now, invested in the chase and possessing the means for making my own determinations, I contributed my share of basic biological findings. What a wonderful adventure, erecting this dusty, dull, dreary, and absolutely indispensable underpinning to inhaled anesthetic pharmacokinetics. From 1961 to 1970, we published 16 reports that incorporated the measurement of solubility. This decreased to two or three reports per decade in subsequent years, most of these in concert with reports on new anesthetics.

Controlling the Concentration at the Effect Site

The early approaches to describing the partial pressure of anesthetic in the brain (or wherever the anesthetic acted) were predicated on the assumption of a constant inspired anesthetic concentration. The answer typically took the form of a curve showing the ratio of F_A (the fraction of anesthetic in the alveoli) to F_I (the fraction of anesthetic in the inspired gas) over time. But that isn't how anesthesia is given. Experienced anesthesiologists know how to administer an anesthetic with high concentrations initially, to achieve a nearly immediate effect. After that, the inspired concentration is quickly reduced, as the anesthesiologist precisely titrates the amount of anesthetic required for the suppression of the response to the surgical stimulus. A sustained constant alveolar (end-tidal) anesthetic concentration provides a closer approximation to the clinical delivery of inhaled anesthetics than delivery of a constant inspired anesthetic concentration. In 1963, Neri Guadagni and I reported on this approach with halothane.[9]

Holding the alveolar concentration constant got closer to a constant anesthetic state than did the application of a constant inspired concentration. However, to be useful, the alveolar concentration had to be reflected in the effect site in the central nervous system, wherever that unknown site might be. This required allowing sufficient time to transfer anesthetic from lungs to site. We could get closer to a constant anesthetic state if we could impose a sustained anesthetizing concentration at the effect site. We didn't know how to do that, in part because we didn't know where that site was (it turned out that for some anesthetics, it wasn't even the brain).[10,11] And, besides, how would we sample the anesthetic at that site? Brain samples were certainly not going to be approved in patients (or anyone else).

It had been known for decades that inhaled anesthetics affected the electroencephalogram.[12,13] Based on this work, Albert Faulconer suggested that we use EEG waveforms as surrogate measures of anesthetic concentration at the effect site. We demonstrated this for ether in the 1960s.[14] Years later, Chris Hull,[15] a British anesthesiologist, and Lewis Sheiner,[16] a clinical pharmacologist at UCSF, worked out the mathematics of characterizing plasma—effect site equilibration rates for muscle relaxants. The effect site is one of the fundamental concepts in anesthetic pharmacology. Decades later, the EEG became a standard clinical monitor of the effect of inhaled and intravenous anesthetics and sedatives on the brain.[17]

Cardiorespiratory Changes Affect Kinetics

We quantified the effects of changes in ventilation and cardiac output on the rate of rise in the alveolar anesthetic concentration.[18,19] It is obvious that an increase in alveolar ventilation delivers more anesthetic to the lungs and thereby accelerates the rise. However, as I discovered in 1956 after hearing John Severinghaus explain it, it is less obvious that increased solubility decreases the rate of rise. It is also less obvious why alterations in ventilation minimally affect the acceleration of poorly soluble anesthetics such as nitrous oxide but greatly affect the acceleration of highly soluble anesthetics such as ether.

Why does solubility play such a profound role? F_A/F_I rapidly increases with poorly soluble anesthetics since little of what is delivered to the lungs is removed. As an extreme case, consider inhaling a substance with no solubility in body tissues at all. After a few breaths to wash in the inspired substance, F_A equals F_I. Even if the patient stops breathing after these first few breaths, F_A continues to equal F_I. This is why, for poorly soluble anesthetics, F_A quickly rises toward and only slowly falls from F_I, even if ventilation is depressed. An increase in ventilation cannot have much effect since F_A quickly rises toward F_I under any circumstances. Conversely, blood absorbs most of a highly soluble anesthetic delivered to the lungs and would do so even if normal ventilation were doubled. Alveolar concentration is proportional to the concentration in blood. With a very soluble anesthetic, doubling ventilation approximately doubles the rise in alveolar concentration until equilibrium is approached.

In contrast to the effect of increasing ventilation, increasing cardiac output hinders the rise in alveolar concentration. As with the effect of changes in ventilation, a change in cardiac output has little effect on the alveolar concentration for poorly soluble anesthetics and a larger, even proportional effect for highly soluble anesthetics. Mathematically, the capacity for anesthetic transport is the product of cardiac output and solubility. That is why they are interchangeable. If you understand one, you understand both.

Anesthetics may depress ventilation, circulation, or both.[20-22] There is some safety when anesthetics depress ventilation and the patient is spontaneously breathing. As breathing slows, the rate of rise in anesthetic concentration also slows, particularly for the more soluble anesthetics as explained above. Anesthetic-induced depression of ventilation creates negative feedback limiting the rise in anesthetic concentration. Thus, spontaneous ventilation increases the safety of inhaled anesthetics.[23] Adding further to the safety of spontaneous ventilation, anesthetic-induced depression of ventilation increases $PaCO_2$, which in turn increases cardiac output.[24,25]

As explained above, the increase in cardiac output decreases the rate of rise of alveolar anesthetic concentration, limiting cardiovascular depression. Conversely, using mechanical ventilation to sustain a normal $PaCO_2$ bypasses this potentially important safety feedback loop, leading to concentration-related depression of cardiac output.[21,26] Anesthetic depression of circulation decreases uptake, hastening the rise of F_A/F_I. The increased F_A further depresses cardiac output, further increasing F_A/F_I. This positive feedback loop can lead to cardiovascular collapse and death.[23] Changes in cardiac output also affect the distribution of anesthetics into peripheral tissues,[18] a complex pharmacokinetic feedback system that is necessarily described by differential equations.

The interactions of solubility, ventilation, cardiac output, anesthetic concentration, and its uptake are more complex than these introductory comments imply. For example, consider a subject inspiring a low concentration of a highly soluble anesthetic. Ignoring the effects on CO_2, doubling ventilation in this subject will double alveolar and (thus) arterial concentrations. Now let's consider the same subject breathing an intermediate concentration of the same highly soluble anesthetic. Again, ignoring the effects on CO_2, if ventilation is doubled then the alveolar concentration more than doubles. The reason is that the uptake of anesthetic will draw more air and anesthetic into the lungs. Almost paradoxically, ventilation more than doubles. Add to these thoughts the effect of the fresh gas inflow rate. A lower fresh gas inflow rate limits the effects of increased ventilation since more gas is rebreathed and uptake has depleted the anesthetic from the rebreathed gases, limiting the capacity of anesthetic uptake to enhance ventilation.

Further complicating matters, surgical stimulation increases both ventilation (in the spontaneously breathing patient) and cardiac output. This antagonizes the ventilatory and circulatory depression caused by inhaled anesthetics.[27,28] In the study by France and colleagues,[28] surgical stimulation increased both alveolar ventilation and production of carbon dioxide, without materially changing $PaCO_2$ at a given target MAC value (1.0, 1.5, or 2.0 MAC). This indicates that surgical stimulation increased metabolism, ventilation, and cardiac output concurrently and to approximately the same extent. As noted in the succeeding paragraph, such concurrent increases can increase F_A/F_I: proportional increases in both cardiac output and ventilation have opposing effects that might exactly oppose each other were it not for the effect of increased cardiac output on tissue time constants.

To explain this, I need to introduce the three concepts: tissue volume, tissue flow, and the time constant. Tissue volume is the capacity of a tissue to hold anesthetic, calculated as anesthetic solubility in the tissue times tissue mass. Tissue flow is total blood flow to the tissue. The time constant is the tissue volume divided by flow. Volume and flow can be expressed for the total tissue, as just described, or per unit of tissue mass. It does not matter; the time constant is the same.

The time constant is the time it takes for a 63% change in tissue concentration following a step change in blood concentration. If cardiac output increases the flow of anesthetic to tissues, then the time constants (volume/flow) for the tissues will decrease. This decrease in the tissue time constant increases the rate at which tissues come into equilibrium with the arterial concentration. This accelerates the rate of rise in F_A/F_I.

This seems paradoxical! Didn't I explain a few paragraphs ago that an increase in cardiac output slows the rate of rise in F_A/F_I? Yes, but, as they say, it's complex. The net effect of increased cardiac output is slower rise in F_A/F_I. However, the effect of increasing uptake from the lungs with increasing cardiac output is slightly offset by the more rapid rise to steady state in peripheral tissues based on the smaller (shorter) time constants.

Stimulation did not change F_A in the study by France and colleagues[28] because the F_A was controlled at targeted levels by altering the delivered concentration of anesthetic.

What If Ventilation, Blood Flow, and Flow Distribution Change Concurrently?

Most of the previous discussion considered the effect of changes in ventilation or changes in circulation independent of each other. But these often occur concurrently. In perhaps the simplest case, assume that ventilation and cardiac output increase in proportion to each other; if ventilation doubles or triples, so does cardiac output. Further, assume that the increases in blood flow occur proportionately in all tissues: if blood flow to the heart doubles, so does blood flow to all other tissues. What then happens to the rise in F_A/F_I? It would be easy to be misled into thinking that the answer is "nothing." That is not correct. Consider the extreme case in which ventilation and cardiac output are both infinitely fast. In that case, F_A/F_I rises instantly from 0 to 1 the moment the anesthetic delivery starts. As a physiologically plausible example, consider a doubling of ventilation and cardiac output. A doubling of ventilation initially doubles delivery of anesthetic to the lungs. If cardiac output doubles, that doubles the blood passing the lungs that removes anesthetic. However, while the doubling of cardiac output initially offsets the doubling of ventilation, it hastens delivery of anesthetic to tissues (exactly as increasing ventilation hastens delivery of anesthesia to the lungs). A doubling of blood flow to a tissue approximately halves the time for equilibration of anesthetic with the tissue, thereby returning increasingly greater concentrations of anesthetic to the lungs. The greater blood flow cannot compensate for the greater delivery of anesthetic by ventilation and the rate of rise in F_A/F_I must increase.[29] This simplest case may explain what happens to F_A/F_I when metabolism increases in febrile patients or perhaps hyperthyroid patients. Metabolism, CO_2 production in all tissues, ventilation, and blood flow increase in rough proportion (ignoring differential blood flows needed to manage temperature regulation).

Nature provides a satisfying experiment testing the above hypothesis. Proportionate increases in ventilation, cardiac output, and the distribution of blood flow per kg of tissue occur with decreasing size of animals. The rat has a greater ventilation and cardiac output per kg than a human. Thus, the rate of increase in F_A/F_I should be more rapid in a rat than a human, and more rapid in a human than a whale. Wahrenbrock and others showed that this was the case.[30]

Under some conditions, the proportional changes in blood flow assumed in previous paragraphs are not found. Ventilation and cardiac output may both double, but the increased cardiac output may not be proportionately increased to all tissues, being more than doubled for some and less for others. This can variously affect the rate of increase in F_A/F_I. In the extreme case of hypovolemic shock, cerebral blood flow is preserved at the expense of blood flow to everything else. In this reduced heart-brain circuit, F_A/F_I rises extremely fast, raising considerable risk of cardiovascular collapse and death.

In the very young patient, the vessel rich group (VRG) of tissues (which include the brain, heart, splanchnic bed, kidney, and endocrine glands) constitutes a greater fraction of body mass, has a greater metabolic rate, and receives a greater blood flow than in the older patient.[29] Although ventilation and cardiac output may be proportionately greater per kg of tissue in the young patient (ie, both ventilation and cardiac output might be 30% greater in the young), two factors lead to a faster rise in F_A/F_I in the younger patient. First, as when the increased blood flow is distributed proportionately to all tissues, the greater blood flow in the young patient accelerates the equilibrium of tissue and blood anesthetic partial pressures (shortens the time constant for tissue equilibration) and thus uptake slows more rapidly in the young, increasing the rate of rise of F_A/F_I. Second, the increase in cardiac output is not proportionately distributed. The brain and other VRG tissues are bigger relative to other tissues in the young. They receive a greater fraction of the cardiac output. The brain and other VRG tissues normally equilibrate quickly with time constants of 3 or 4 minutes in adults and even shorter time constants in the young. Because these tissues receive a greater fraction of the cardiac output in children, their rapid equilibration results in a more rapid rise in blood concentration, which hastens the rise of F_A/F_I.

The above argument indicates a more rapid induction of anesthesia in the young. And the smaller functional residual capacity in the younger patient would accelerate the equilibration of the gases in the lung, adding further to the speed of induction. The increased fraction of cardiac output delivered to the brain decreases the time constant for blood-brain equilibration, further speeding induction of anesthesia. If the inspired concentration is not increased, the higher MAC values in young patients[31,32] might slightly offset the faster equilibration kinetics. Even if the same inspired concentration is used in young and older patients, induction is usually more rapid in the young patient.

In the above example, children have a proportionate increase in regional blood flow to rapidly equilibrating tissues, which increases the rate of increase in F_A/F_I and thus the rate of anesthetic induction. The opposite situation will occur if, instead, there is an increase in regional blood flow to muscle or (especially) fat, which have huge capacity to store anesthetic. These tissues equilibrate very slowly. Even though these tissues will equilibrate more quickly if they receive a greater fraction of cardiac output, that will not compensate for the slower equilibration in brain and other rapidly equilibrating tissues because of fractionally reduced blood flow. The net effect of a proportional increase in blood flow to muscle and fat will be to slow the rise of F_A/F_I and the onset of anesthesia.

Consider the case of an increase in cardiac output matched by a proportional increase in ventilation, but with a redistribution of cardiac output to muscle (eg, exercise). The net effect might be a slower increase in F_A/F_I because a significant fraction of the drug taken up from the lungs is dumped into a muscle sink.[33] For a time, uptake is increased, and thereby the rate of rise of F_A/F_I slows. Excitation on induction of anesthesia might supply circumstances leading to an increased blood flow to muscle... and a delay in induction of anesthesia. Similarly, weight reduction or injection of a beta-agonist can increase blood flow to fat.[34] The increased blood flow to fat would be expected to slow the rise of F_A/F_I during induction of anesthesia.

In my clinical practice in the 1960s, I would occasionally anesthetize children. I remember seeing these principles play out when I anesthetized them with ether. I would tell them stories and pretends. "There's a rabbit in the mask that you are going to breathe from and this funny rabbit smells of onions because he eats onions. See if you can smell the rabbit." And the patient and I would see if we could smell the rabbit. I adjusted the gaseous river of highly soluble ether flowing into child's lungs as I maintained the happy deception of the rabbit with halitosis. By and by the child went to sleep. When the child woke he would ask where the rabbit had gone. I don't think I ever explained that the rabbit had vanished into thin (and expired) air.

Body Temperature Can Affect the Rate of Anesthetic Induction

A decrease in body temperature influences both pharmacokinetics and pharmacodynamics of inhaled anesthetics, increasingly delaying induction of anesthesia as anesthetic solubility increases.[35] Consider the changes in pharmacodynamics. MAC rectilinearly decreases for potent clinical anesthetics as temperature decreases.[36,37] One might think that if the patient is cold, then the decrease in MAC with colder temperature would result in a more rapid onset of anesthetic effect. However, as is so often the case, it is more complicated.

Pharmacokinetics also change with decreasing temperature. For starters, decreasing body temperature increases the solubility of anesthetics in the brain and other tissues.[38] As we know, increased solubility slows the onset of anesthesia. Decreasing temperatures also decrease metabolism, which decreases both ventilation and cardiac output. A decrease in ventilation slows the delivery of anesthetic to the lungs, and a decrease in perfusion slows the delivery of anesthetic to the brain and other tissues, but it may increase the rate of rise of F_A/F_I because uptake from the alveoli decreases.

However, it gets more complex still. Not only does solubility increase in the brain, it increases in the blood. This slows the rate of rise of the anesthetic partial pressure in blood. However, the blood has more capacity to deliver anesthetic to the brain. The significantly reduced cerebral oxygen requirements with hypothermia will reduce cerebral blood flow, overall decreasing anesthetic delivery.

The net result is that induction of anesthesia slows as body temperature decreases. If the cold patient is given the same inspired concentration as a normothermic patient, the eventual anesthetic state will be more profound in the cold patient. However, the slowing of induction differs among anesthetics as a function of solubility. A more soluble anesthetic will have greater delay in induction consequent to a decrease in temperature than a less soluble anesthetic.[35] Fortunately, this is mostly an intellectual exercise because our patients typically come to us at 37°.

Ventilation/Perfusion Inequalities

The usefulness of the F_A/F_I ratio depends on the partial pressure fraction in arterial blood, F_a, closely following the partial pressure fraction in the alveoli, F_A. Unfortunately, F_A-F_a differences do appear in normal subjects, particularly early in anesthesia.[39] For nitrous oxide, the differences become minimal within a half hour of breathing a constant F_I.[39]

F_A-F_a differences become clinically important in the presence of ventilation/perfusion (V/Q) mismatch. V/Q mismatch may occur with diseases such as emphysema, atelectasis, pneumonia, and pneumothorax, as well as with congenital anomalies. Anesthetics also cause V/Q mismatch through bronchodilation, evidenced by the increase in the gradient for arterial to end-tidal gas for CO_2 (the a-A gradient) seen with induction of anesthesia. Common interventions such as muscle paralysis and mechanical ventilation cause some V/Q mismatch.

A more extreme case is endobronchial intubation (placement of the tracheal tube into a main bronchus), which results in ventilation confined to the left or right lung. The ventilated lung gets twice the normal ventilation, while the other lung isn't ventilated at all. The nonventilated lung is still perfused. Since no anesthetic is delivered, no anesthetic is taken up by the blood perfusing that lung. F_A, as measured using end-tidal concentrations, and F_a, the arterial concentration, will diverge.[40]

Not surprisingly, the divergence of alveolar and arterial concentration with endobronchial intubation (or V/Q mismatch generally) is a function of solubility. Consider a poorly soluble gas, such as nitrous oxide or cyclopropane. For such drugs, the rate of rise of F_A/F_I is primarily determined by the rate of equilibration with the inspired gas, not by systemic uptake from the lungs. (Consider the extreme case of an insoluble gas. The rate of rise of F_A/F_I would be entirely determined by the rate of washin from the breathing circuit.) As a result, for a poorly soluble gas, following endobronchial intubation end-tidal increase in partial pressure would not deviate greatly from normal. F_A, measured in the ventilated lung, is primarily determined by washin from the circuit. Increasing ventilation cannot increase F_A to more than F_I. As a result, increasing ventilation to one lung cannot compensate for not ventilating the other lung at all for a poorly soluble anesthetic. The result is that for a poorly soluble anesthetic the arterial partial pressure initially would be approximately half normal.[40]

Now consider how these factors affect equilibrium with a highly soluble anesthetic such as ether or methoxyflurane. The nonventilated lung doesn't get anesthetic, but the ventilated lung gets nearly twice as much. Doubling the ventilation approximately doubles the delivery and thus doubles the concentration—the partial pressure—of anesthetic in blood. Such a doubling almost completely compensates for the absence of ventilation in the remaining lung. Thus, the rate of increase in anesthetic partial pressure in arterial blood is unaffected, not delayed by the ventilation/perfusion inequality.[40] Using dogs and humans,[41] Stoelting and Longnecker confirmed these predictions.

This is analogous to the effect of one-lung ventilation on PaO_2 and $PaCO_2$. Oxygen is poorly soluble. As a result, one-lung ventilation can't compensate for the lack of any oxygen delivery to the other lung and may easily lead to hypoxemia. However, CO_2 is highly soluble. If the ventilated lung receives a nearly normal tidal volume, then a nearly normal amount of CO_2 will be removed from the blood perfusing the ventilated lung. That is why hypoxemia is a grave risk with one-lung ventilation, while hypercarbia is rarely a problem.

All Models Are Wrong

The model of anesthetic uptake and distribution presented at the 1962 conference by Mackrell, Mapleson, Price, and Severinghaus, and extended by my work, was obviously correct in concept, wasn't it? It rested on the findings of myriad scientists about anatomy, physiology, chemistry, and physics. The model described how gases drawn into the alveoli quickly moved into the passing blood, with equilibration rapidly established between alveolar and arterial anesthetic partial pressures. The anesthetic in arterial blood differentially distributed into tissues as a function of perfusion and solubility. For the model to match experimental observations, the model required that body tissues be divided into three groups: the vessel rich group (VRG), the muscle group (MG), and the fat group (FG). A fourth tissue group, the vessel poor group (VPG; eg, bone, ligaments, tendons, cartilage, hair) could be ignored because it received no appreciable perfusion and thus could not affect uptake.

For me, but not for the other investigators, this model also predicted the effect of inspired concentration (the concentration and second gas effects). And the predictions of the model followed our experimental data. The model provided a framework to understand how cardiorespiratory variations, temperature changes, ventilation/perfusion inequalities, and inspired concentration affected uptake and distribution.

As mentioned above, Perl and colleagues,[42] supported by Rackow and colleagues,[43] questioned whether another factor, intertissue diffusion, affected F_A/F_I. For example, could a drug move directly from the vessel-rich group to the fat group? If so, our model would not account for this because our model lacked intertissue diffusion. Nitrous oxide and cyclopropane supposedly had nearly identical blood/gas partition coefficients. If other lean tissues also had similar partition coefficients for cyclopropane and nitrous oxide, then the F_A/F_I for these anesthetics should increase at similar rates. But Rackow and colleagues found that the F_A/F_I for cyclopropane increased about 5% more slowly than for nitrous oxide. He accounted for this discrepancy by modifying the model to include diffusion of cyclopropane from well-perfused tissues (eg, intestine or kidney) to adjacent (mesenteric, omental, perirenal) fat.

HL Menckens observed that "there is always a well-known solution to every human problem—neat, plausible, and wrong."[44] I both had it wrong and right. Eventually we determined that Rackow's results were the result of breaking the law—Henry's law. Henry's law states that the content of gas in a liquid after equilibration with that same gas in a gas mixture is proportional to the partial pressure of the gas in the gas mixture. Nitrous oxide follows Henry's law in the blood. That means that the concentration of nitrous oxide in a liquid equilibrated with 80% nitrous oxide in air is eight times more than the concentration of nitrous oxide in a liquid equilibrated with 10% nitrous oxide in air. Lockhart also found that isoflurane and halothane follow Henry's law in the brain.[45] Henry's law allows us to make assumptions about the content of anesthetic in blood based on observations of the partial pressure of the anesthetic in exhaled gas.

Unfortunately, cyclopropane does not follow Henry's law in blood, as Gregory and I demonstrated.[46] Cyclopropane avidly binds to hemoglobin. The hemoglobin binding sites fill up at fairly low cyclopropane concentrations, becoming saturated at cyclopropane concentrations well below 100%. The result is that at 1% concentration, cyclopropane has a blood/gas partition coefficient of 0.6, reflecting the high binding to hemoglobin. At 100% cyclopropane, the cyclopropane blood/gas partition coefficient might be 0.47.

Perl assumed that the blood/gas partition coefficients for cyclopropane and nitrous oxide were 0.42 and 0.47, respectively. Rackow drew his conclusions based on the same assumptions. His experiment used 0.5% inspired cyclopropane and 4% inspired nitrous oxide, without accounting for the greater cyclopropane blood/gas partition coefficient at 0.5% inspired concentration. To his credit, he did consider the possibility of a violation of Henry's law, "Changing only the blood/air partition coefficient of cyclopropane…from 0.47 to 0.61…is implausible (it isn't) and in any event corrects the discrepancy only over a short time interval (apparently 5 to 30 minutes)." Not only was it not implausible, it proved to explain his findings. If myoglobin acted like hemoglobin, that, too, undermined the implausible argument.

Science is asymptotic. Subsequent observations demonstrated that Rackow's and Perl's intuition about intertissue diffusion was correct. Intertissue diffusion indeed played a role. In the 1980s, Randy Carpenter and I tested whether a four-compartment model (lungs, VRG, MG, and FG) could explain data from measurement of the washin and washout of inhaled anesthetics in humans.[47,48] To test this, we needed far more observations than had been collected in the past. In particular, if the fat group were important, we would need to measure anesthetic partial pressure in venous blood over the course of days to observe the washout of drug from the large reservoir in body fat. Even the effect of the muscle group would require measurements over many hours. That problem wasn't insurmountable because we did not have to rely on washin measurements alone; we could test change during several days of washout. And, indeed, that is what we did in several succeeding studies.

For precisely 2 hours we measured the washin of enflurane, halothane, isoflurane, or methoxyflurane given in a background of nitrous oxide and oxygen simultaneously to nine healthy (other than the surgical condition) normocapnic surgical patients.[47] Ventilation was adjusted to maintain normal PCO_2 (normocapnia). Each potent anesthetic was given at a sub-MAC concentration with a total inspired concentration of 1.1 MAC. We ceased administering the potent anesthetics after 2 hours, maintaining anesthesia for ongoing surgery with nitrous oxide and intravenous agents. We measured the partial pressure of the potent anesthetics in venous blood for 5 to 9 days. We fit polyexponential models to the washin and washout data using successively more exponents (compartments) for each anesthetic for each patient (36 data sets). In 27 of the 36 data sets, the best fit was obtained with a five-compartment model.[47] At worst, the resulting hybrid rate constants were within a factor of 3 or 4 of what might have been predicted for the lungs, VRG, MG, and FG, closest for the longer rate constants (eg, within 35% for the FG). Changing the duration of anesthesia did not alter the results. Giving the four anesthetics for 30 minutes rather than 2 hours produced the same findings.[48] Similar studies in pigs in 1990 (for desflurane, sevoflurane, isoflurane and halothane)[49] and in humans in 1991 (sevoflurane with isoflurane[50]; and desflurane, with isoflurane and halothane[51]) consistently found that a five-compartment model best predicted the results. We found similar results in older patients.[52]

One of our coinvestigators in this work was Argyro ("Rula") Fassoulaki, a visiting professor from Athens. Rula was a smart lady for whom English was a second language. She was still learning her way about the laboratory when she spilled a bottle of acetone on a countertop. The acetone immediately caught fire! Our chief technician, Brynte Johnson, shouted "*Rula! Alert!*" as he quickly quenched the flame. Rula was puzzled: "*What is a Lert?*"

Returning to the need for five tissue compartments to adequately describe our data, what was this "fifth compartment," this additional tissue group with a time constant of approximately 500 minutes, a substantial tissue group that accounted for perhaps 30% of the anesthetic taken up? No other known tissue group, except possibly the fat in bone marrow, has the blood flow and solubility that the time constant demanded. However, this was a large compartment, and there isn't enough bone marrow to explain how it could account for approximately 30% of the anesthetic taken up. Bone marrow might have accounted for 7% or 8%, but not 30%.

As Perl and Rackow had done before us, we speculated that this tissue group was fat juxtaposed to highly perfused tissues, with the fat receiving anesthetic by intertissue diffusion. Our speculation was experimentally demonstrated by others using autoradiographs, which directly showed that anesthetic is transferred from the kidney to perirenal fat by intertissue diffusion.[53]

Duration and Concentration Affects Kinetics

In the previous section, we found that increasing the duration of anesthesia did not change how anesthetics distribute within the body. Our five-compartment model described anesthetic distribution for both a half-hour and a 2-hour anesthetic experience. The tissue compartments were the lung, VRG, MG, FG, and ITDG (inter-tissue diffusion group). The model captured the accumulation of anesthetic over time in the body compartments. The model accounted for the observation that the more soluble the anesthetic in body tissue, the longer it took for the tissue to equilibrate. With highly soluble volatile anesthetics, the time constants of the FG and ITDG are so small that it would take days of anesthesia to reach steady state. With soluble volatile anesthetics, at typical anesthetic durations, the MG, FG, and ITDG do not reach steady state, accumulating in tissues only until the delivery of anesthetic is discontinued at the end of the procedure. The result is that the longer an anesthetic is delivered, and the higher the anesthetic concentration, the longer it will take for the body to eliminate the anesthetic at the end of the procedure. This explains the clinically obvious observation that patients awaken quickly from brief anesthetics, even with highly soluble anesthetics, and very slowly from long anesthetics, especially with more soluble anesthetics. It also explains the rapid washout of nitrous oxide, where the compartments equilibrate quickly, and slow washout of halothane, where the compartments equilibrate slowly.[54]

This study of washout in dogs by my research fellow, Bob Stoelting, and me required establishment of whole-body equilibration, something that might take a combination of overpressure and prolonged (eg, ≥24 hours) anesthetic delivery, especially with the highly soluble, slowly acting methoxyflurane. To expedite induction of anesthesia we initially gave the rapid-acting cyclopropane and then converted to methoxyflurane anesthesia for the prolonged equilibration. On one occasion, Bob was charged with setting up the anesthetic system for induction and maintenance while I attended to some matter in my office. He called me after the dog had been prepared for the study. I ran up to the lab, and we began the induction. Bob held the mask firmly over the dog's muzzle and turned on a flow of cyclopropane sufficient to induce anesthesia in a small elephant. I held the less dangerous but smellier end of the dog. Rather than succumbing to the effect of the cyclopropane, the dog became increasingly agitated, supplying generous amounts of urine and feces. Bob cranked up the cyclopropane, enough to stun a medium-sized elephant. From my southern vantage point, I noticed that Bob had not attached a rebreathing bag to the anesthetic circuit. Our poor dog was breathing mostly room air and sufficient cyclopropane to enter the excitement phase of anesthesia. Perhaps because I was struggling with dog poop, I yelled "You idiot!" and pointed to the absence of the bag. Bob, who is not an idiot, says no one has called him that since. However, he's never forgotten to attach the rebreathing bag since.

Solubility Is Everything

Because duration of anesthesia and delivered concentration determine the anesthetic partial pressure in tissues, they influence the partial pressure of anesthetic in the blood returning to the lungs and thus influence the rate of recovery from anesthesia.[37,55] At anesthetizing concentrations and greater, the time required for emergence from anesthesia increases with increasing MAC-hours of anesthetic delivery.[55]

The solubility of anesthetic in blood determines the steepness of the slope relating MAC-hours to the time needed for recovery—ie, a greater solubility produces a steeper slope and a lower solubility produce a flatter slope[55]—a reasonable result that follows from where the beginning and end must be with highly soluble versus poorly soluble anesthetics. For sufficiently small MAC-hours of anesthesia, awakening will be rapid regardless of solubility. Anesthetic effect site concentrations in the lightly anesthetized patient lie not far above the line separating unconsciousness and consciousness. As the MAC-hours and thus the accumulated stores of anesthetic increase, an increase in solubility slows the rate at which the stores can leave the body, and thus slows the rate at which the line can be reached and awakening can occur.

We first turned to rats to document the importance of anesthetic duration on the rate of recovery.[55] We followed this with studies in adult humans anesthetized for 2, 4, or 8 hours with 1.25 MAC desflurane versus sevoflurane.[56] Elimination during the first hour of recovery occurs 40% more rapidly with the less soluble desflurane and accompanies a more rapid recovery of cerebral function such as speed of return of response to command (**Figure 8.1**). These are similar to the findings in children anesthetized with desflurane versus isoflurane.[57]

The clinical implications of solubility are often misunderstood. It is tempting to believe that poorly soluble drugs such as nitrous oxide are appropriate for brief cases, while more soluble anesthetics, and hence "slower" drugs, are more suitable for longer cases. Similarly, the less soluble desflurane might be considered a drug for brief outpatient procedures, while the more soluble sevoflurane might be considered more appropriate for longer inpatient procedures. However, this is not what the pharmacokinetics suggest. The pharmacokinetics show that for brief procedures it makes almost no difference what drug you use. With little time for drugs to accumulate in body tissues, emergence from any of the inhaled anesthetics will be rapid. Less soluble anesthetics are primarily of use in very long cases. Drug accumulation in peripheral tissues can profoundly slow emergence after very long exposures. The more soluble the anesthetic, the more

Time from Cessation of Anesthesia to Response to Command
and to Orientation to Place and Date

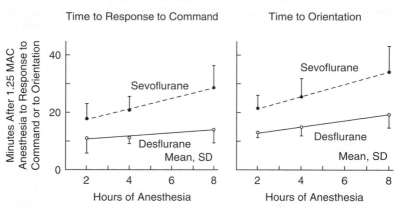

Figure 8.1   For a given duration of anesthesia in volunteers, the time to response to command (eg, "open your eyes") or orientation to date and time took nearly twice as long after anesthesia with the more soluble sevoflurane (blood/gas partition coefficient 0.65) than after anesthesia with desflurane (blood/gas partition coefficient 0.45). (From Eger EIII, Gong D, Koblin DD, et al. Effect of anesthetic duration on kinetic and recovery characteristics of desflurane vs. sevoflurane (plus compound A) in volunteers. *Anesth Analg.* 1998;86:414-421.)

drug accumulates in tissue with prolonged administration. Thus, less soluble anesthetics show minimal benefits for short anesthetics, but may appreciably hasten recovery following long anesthetics. It is my impression that many of my colleagues have this exactly backwards.

Our work in the 1960s created a mathematical model that described the behavior of inhaled anesthetics. Our model was anchored in basic experimental observations of solubilities and physiology. It predicted how anesthetics would behave in clinical work, but it would take years for our predictions to be tested.

Decades later, I helped Rachel McKay and her collaborators demonstrate the potential clinical importance of the delay in recovery with increasing solubility and anesthetic duration.[58] She studied otherwise healthy patients randomly assigned to have anesthesia maintained with either desflurane or sevoflurane. The attending anesthetist determined the concentration of anesthetic to be delivered. Overall, the anesthetics did not differ in duration or MAC. The observer determining the awakening time was blinded to the anesthetic selection.

McKay and her colleagues determined that patients given the less soluble anesthetic, desflurane, awoke more rapidly in several ways. One was the standard test of the time to awakening to command ("Open your eyes"). A finding with implications for patient safety was that patients given desflurane recovered the capacity to swallow 20 mL of water without coughing or drooling sooner than those given sevoflurane (**Figure 8.2**). Furthermore, the time from discontinuation of anesthetic administration to swallowing water without coughing or drooling was shorter after desflurane and correlated significantly with MAC-hours of anesthesia with sevoflurane but not with desflurane. McKay and colleagues also found that the time to swallowing water without coughing or drooling increased with increasing body mass index (BMI) for patients given sevoflurane but not those given desflurane.

The study by Rachel McKay and her colleagues demonstrates the role of solubility implied by the mathematical models of uptake and distribution. Specifically, various measures of recovery support the finding that decreased solubility results in faster offset of anesthetic drug effect, and that physiologic changes that might delay emergence, such as increased BMI, will have greater effect on recovery from more soluble anesthetics.

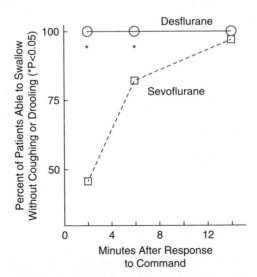

Figure 8.2 Patients randomized to identical MAC hours of desflurane or sevoflurane responded to command sooner after discontinuation of desflurane, with earlier control of swallowing. (Adapted from McKay RE, Malhotra A, Cakmakkaya OS, Hall KT, McKay WR, Apfel CC. Effect of increased body mass index and anesthetic duration on recovery of protective airway reflexes after sevoflurane vs desflurane. *Br J Anaesth.* 2010;104:175-182.)

Metabolism Can Affect Kinetics

The metabolism of injected drugs such as midazolam, propofol, and fentanyl affects their pharmacokinetics and clinical use in complex manners, as Larry Saidman and I demonstrated for thiopental.[59,60] Similarly, the degradation of inhaled anesthetics by metabolism or by carbon dioxide absorbents in rebreathing circuits has implications for their safety, pharmacokinetics, and clinical delivery. Degradation products can be toxic. For example, sevoflurane is degraded by soda lime or Baralyme into the Compound A.[61] Desflurane is slightly degraded by desiccated soda lime or Baralyme into carbon monoxide.[62] Soda lime degrades some experimental anesthetics (eg, CHF_2-O-CH$(CF_3)_2$) so rapidly—in seconds—that these anesthetics cannot be delivered in a rebreathing circuit containing the absorbent (Eger, unpublished data).

Some anesthetics undergo extensive metabolism, usually by the liver. Halsey and friends studied the hepatic metabolism of anesthetics in miniature swine.[63] Methoxyflurane and halothane underwent approximately 50% and 35% metabolism, respectively. Enflurane had significantly less metabolism, just 10%, and isoflurane and cyclopropane were not metabolized at all. These results suggested that for drugs like halothane, metabolism might play a significant role in uptake, distribution, and recovery. Our model didn't anticipate this. We missed an important finding!

It turns out that halothane metabolism isn't proportional to halothane concentration. For most drugs, if you double the concentration, you double the rate of hepatic metabolism. However, for some drugs, most famously alcohol, the body has very limited metabolic capacity. Once alcohol concentrations rise high enough to saturate metabolism, increasing alcohol concentration does not increase metabolism. Sawyer and colleagues found that at trace halothane concentrations, nearly 100% of the halothane passing through the liver underwent metabolism.[64] However, hepatic metabolism quickly becomes saturated. At just 0.01% MAC, the liver clears 50% of the halothane delivered to it. At anesthetic concentrations, the liver metabolizes a trivial fraction of the halothane. Thus, there was an aspect of our model that was wrong, but only at trivial concentrations that were not important in understanding halothane uptake and distribution during anesthesia. Bullet dodged!

We followed up on this observation. In a single test swine, Sawyer and I found the same change from first-order (ie, dose-proportional) pharmacokinetics to zero-order (ie, saturable) pharmacokinetics with increasing concentrations of the anesthetic fluroxene.[65] High concentrations, concentrations approaching MAC, saturated the capacity to metabolize fluroxene. Using different techniques, Hitt and colleagues found similar results for enflurane in rats.[66]

A study in humans by Cahalan and colleagues found that a similar low halothane concentration, roughly 1/30th of MAC, resulted in 50% metabolism.[67] Consistent with these data, White and colleagues found that rats metabolized a greater fraction of enflurane or methoxyflurane when these anesthetics were given for the same MAC-hours at low concentrations (for a longer time) than at greater concentrations (for a shorter time).[68] One clinical implication is that a lack of metabolite toxicity from a given duration (MAC-hours) of general anesthesia does not necessarily mean that the same MAC-hours at subanesthetic concentrations would lack toxicity from metabolites.

As our model grew with these additional observations, we understood that the role of metabolism changed depending on the duration and dose administered. Specifically, the amount of anesthetic taken up per unit time decreases with increasing duration of anesthesia as saturation of lean tissues occurs. Once anesthesia has been administered for an hour or so, the lean tissue is saturated, and most uptake is by slowly equilibrating fat. Since the time constant for uptake by fat is measured in days, even prolonged anesthesia does not produce a substantial partial pressure of anesthetic in fat. However, because volatile anesthetics are so soluble in fat, the absolute amount of anesthetic in fat can be substantial after prolonged administration of anesthetics. This large store is released during recovery. Much of it will be released at trace concentrations, meaning that it will be subjected to a greater metabolism than if it were released at clinical concentrations. An implication of our expanded model was the finding that metabolism as a percentage of halothane uptake decreases as the dose increases. Conversely, at clinically relevant doses, increased duration of halothane administration increases the fraction of anesthetic subject to metabolism.

I pursued the relationship between dose and metabolism in clinical studies with Michael Cahalan and colleagues.[69] We measured the time required for clinical recovery at different concentrations of inspired enflurane or halothane following 2-hour exposure to these anesthetics. When the enflurane concentration was approximately one-third of MAC, approximately 10% of the anesthetic taken up was metabolized. A fourfold increase in enflurane dose did not change this. However, for halothane, the results were different. At inspired halothane concentrations of one-third of MAC, approximately 55% of the halothane taken up was metabolized. As our model predicted, this decreased (to 41%) when the halothane concentration was increased fourfold.

Our finding helped explain clinical differences between enflurane and halothane. Specifically, the elimination of anesthetic (the rate of decrease of F_A/F_{A0} where F_{A0} is the alveolar concentration immediately before discontinuation of anesthetic administration) is more rapid with halothane than with enflurane.[19,70,71]

We found that this could be explained by the greater metabolism of halothane (30%-50%, vs 3%-8% for enflurane), which played a more important role than the lesser solubility of enflurane in blood and tissues.

One other result flowed from the study conducted by Cahalan and his colleagues.[69] Metabolism of enflurane or halothane was not influenced by the presence or absence of 70% nitrous oxide. For halothane, metabolism was 55%, regardless of whether or not nitrous oxide was administered.

Kinetics and Recovery From Anesthesia

Kinetics dictate the time course of induction of anesthesia. Increased solubility of the inhaled anesthetic slows the rate of increase of F_A/F_I. The anesthesia practitioner must account for this during induction. To achieve rapid onset with more soluble anesthetics, clinicians needed to "overpressure" (start with a higher inspired concentration) to compensate for the slower rate of increase. This may be more obvious if we turn F_A/F_I upside down, ie, to F_I/F_A and require F_A to remain constant—as it does when we keep the anesthetic level constant. A greater solubility demands a greater F_I (a greater overpressure) to hold a given F_A constant.

Nitrous Oxide Can Expand or Pressurize Gas Spaces

Proteins and fat in blood and tissues take up volatile anesthetics just as they take up injected intravenous anesthetics. Drug bound to receptors is in rapid equilibration with the free fraction of both volatile and injected anesthetics and is responsible for pharmacological action. Volatile anesthetics differ from injected intravenous drugs in their capacity to move from blood or a tissue into gas spaces. Appreciable volumes of inhaled anesthetics dissolve in blood if the anesthetic has adequate solubility. If the drug has low potency, and must therefore be given at high partial pressure, the transfer from tissue to gas spaces may be clinically consequential.

Such is the case with nitrous oxide and with a few obsolete (and explosive!) anesthetics (acetylene, cyclopropane, and ethylene). When these gases are transported by blood to tissues containing a closed space filled with a poorly soluble gas (eg, nitrogen), for example, the intestines, the anesthetic gas will quickly equilibrate with the gas in the closed space. If the nitrogen in the closed space moved equally quickly into the blood, then the space would not expand. However, nitrogen is poorly soluble in blood, so the washout of nitrogen is far slower than the washin of anesthetic. Intestinal gas is mostly hydrogen or methane, which are also much less soluble than nitrous oxide.

Our model provides the mathematics of this expansion: 1/(1-fraction inspired gas). For example, if the lungs contain 50% nitrous oxide, then equilibrium with a gas space would result in a twofold expansion (eg, 1/(1-0.5) = 1/0.5 = 2). If the lungs contain 75% nitrous oxide, then equilibrium will occur at a fourfold expansion (eg, 1/(1-0.75) = 1/0.25 = 4). Equilibration occurs almost instantly with air bubbles,[72] requires a few minutes with a pneumothorax,[73] and takes a few hours with intestinal gas.[73,74]

Such an expansion can be highly consequential. Expansion of bowel gas over several hours can impede surgery. This is minor compared to the conversion of a small pneumothorax into a life-threatening tension pneumothorax in a few minutes. The expansion of a gas embolus, even an embolus of carbon dioxide, can increase pulmonary artery pressures 5.5 times more rapidly in the presence of 80% nitrous oxide.[75] An even worse outcome is the expansion of a modest amount of venous air into an air embolus causing circulatory arrest. Thus, our models of uptake and distribution may be more than hypothetical abstractions. They may provide clinical insights essential to the safe use of inhaled anesthetic drugs.

We anesthetists add to the physiological closed gas spaces within the body by our insertion of gas-filled balloons, the cuffs on tracheal tubes,[76] laryngeal mask airways,[77] or the balloons on Swan-Ganz catheters.[78,79] The expansion of such gas-filled spaces may encroach on and damage adjacent tissues, although long-lasting injury is a rare event.

But sometimes noncompliant walls surround a gas space. Consider the air surrounded by the skull in pneumoencephalography (fortunately an obsolete procedure), or the air within a gas bubble injected into the eye. The differential equations describing gas ingress into such spaces predict an increase in pressure rather than expansion in volume. The pressure in the enclosed space at equilibration will be 1 atm plus the partial pressure of the anesthetic gas.[80] For example, if the patient breathes 50% nitrous oxide, the partial pressure at equilibrium would be 1.5 atm (1 atm +0.5 atm from the nitrous oxide in the blood). If this happens to an air bubble in the eye, it will flatten the blood vessels and halt retinal blood flow, potentially causing blindness.[81] Air in the brain ventricles may take 5 days to clear. Expansion of this air from nitrous oxide will cause compression of the brain, possibly compromising cerebral blood flow.[82]

Anesthetic Circuit Structure Influences Kinetics

Anesthetists use rebreathing systems to conserve precious anesthetic vapors and minimize contamination of operating room air with anesthetic. As anesthetics enter the body via the breathing circuit, the kinetics of the breathing circuit influence the rate of onset and offset of anesthesia. The site at which fresh inflowing gases enter the circuit relative to the placement of the inspiratory and expiratory valves determines efficiency of the circle system—the extent to which fresh gas is conserved.[83,84] Modern anesthesia machines are designed to maximally conserve anesthetic vapor.

Effect of Anesthetic Loss Through Skin and Membrane on Uptake

There is another route by which drugs might be lost from the body: direct transfer from the skin to the air. After discovering that metabolism could add an important component of uptake and distribution, we turned to the question of whether anesthetics might be eliminated by direct transfer from the skin. This seemed unlikely because the skin is a superb barrier to transfer in and out of the body. However, we needed to be certain.

To measure direct transfer, we placed the subjects' arm in an air-tight chamber while the subject inhaled an anesthetic. To understand the transfer through the skin, we measured the volume of gas in the chamber, the surface area of skin in the chamber, and the anesthetic partial pressure in the chamber. We also measured the concurrent anesthetic partial pressure in arterial blood. From these data we calculated the rate at which anesthetic gases transferred across the skin into the chamber. We then added transfer through the skin to our mathematical model of anesthetic uptake and distribution. As expected, the loss proved to be minimal, too small to materially affect the rate of anesthetic uptake (F_A/F_I).[85-87] For example, at a steady state inhaled nitrous oxide concentration of 70%, percutaneous loss was 3.6 mL/min/m^2. This is about an order of magnitude less than nitrous oxide uptake during the first hour or two of anesthesia.

By design, the skin is uniquely impermeable. We measured anesthetic transfer across other membranes, membranes that might be exposed to air during surgery, resulting in perioperative loss of anesthetic. In vitro measurements demonstrated a 10- to- 40-fold greater rate of diffusion across the amniotic membrane than across the skin.[88] We found that anesthetics also cross peritoneal and pleural membranes much faster than skin, but slower than amniotic membranes.[89] The amount of drug transferred across peritoneal and pleural membranes correlated with the solubilities of the anesthetic, being four to five times greater (per percent anesthetic) for halothane than for desflurane. Even so, the transfer across these membranes proved too small to materially influence the uptake of inhaled anesthetics.

The Concentration and Second Gas Effects

I fortuitously stumbled across the concentration effect while testing the effect of the inspired concentration on the rate of rise of the alveolar concentration. As I write this, I vaguely remember that I was trying to show that the inspired concentration had no effect on the rate at which F_A/F_I increased. Someone must have told me that it didn't, and I dutifully tried to prove the point. But the more I tried, the more obvious it became that concentration **did** affect the F_A/F_I of the gas whose concentration had been increased. The greater the inspired concentration, the faster the increase in the F_A/F_I ratio. I unimaginatively named this the "concentration effect."

As indicated at the beginning of this chapter, I presented the concentration effect at the 1962 Conference on Anesthetic Uptake and Distribution in New York.[90] It was published the next year.[8] At the meeting, Bob Epstein commented that the concentration effect must also apply to any gas given concurrently. That is, the appreciable uptake of nitrous oxide in the first few minutes of anesthesia would not only increase the rate of rise of the F_A/F_I for nitrous oxide, it must also increase the F_A/F_I for concurrently administered oxygen or that of any other second gas such as an anesthetic. And it would do so for the same reasons that underlie the concentration effect. He called this the "second gas effect."[91]

As explained in Chapter 5, two related factors underlie the concentration and second gas effects. First, there is an increase in inspired volume of gas consequent to the uptake of appreciable volumes of some anesthetic, usually nitrous oxide. Second, there is a concentrating of residual gases by this same appreciable uptake of some anesthetic, usually nitrous oxide.[92] Epstein documented his theory in dogs,[91] and Taheri and I later repeated the documentation in patients.[93]

More than a decade after Epstein's report we invented a simple way to mimic the concentration effect.[94] We knew that, by definition, there could be no concentration effect at trace concentrations of anesthetic: the rate of increase in F_A/F_I would be determined by the balance between anesthetic input by ventilation and its removal by uptake. Anesthetic solubility along with cardiac output and the alveolar-to-venous gradient determined uptake. Thus, all things being equal, F_A/F_I would increase in inverse proportion to anesthetic solubility. At the other extreme, ventilation with 100% of some anesthetic gas, uptake, no matter how large, could not affect the rate of increase in F_A/F_I. Consider why. Inspiration of one breath of 100% of nitrous oxide would produce a concentration equal to the alveolar tidal volume divided by the alveolar tidal volume plus the functional residual capacity. Some of the inspired nitrous oxide would be taken up. Because the lung does not change its structure, the uptake would create a negative pressure that would draw into the lungs a volume of nitrous oxide equal to the volume taken up. The result would be an absence of a change in the concentration of nitrous oxide, no matter how much nitrous oxide might be taken up. Uptake would not influence the rate of increase of F_A/F_I. In sum, at trace concentrations, F_A/F_I would increase at a rate inversely related to solubility, and at 100% inspired concentration, it would increase at a rate independent of solubility.

But what about intervening concentrations? Our model demonstrated that we could mathematically incorporate the concentration effect by changing the blood/gas partition coefficient from λ to λ' where $\lambda' = \lambda \times (1 - F_I)$. thus, if $F_I = 0$, $\lambda' = \lambda$. In this situation, anesthetic uptake (F_A/F_I) is proportional to solubility. But if $F_I = 1.0$ then $\lambda' = 0$. In this setting, F_A/F_I starts at 1 and doesn't change. There is no effect of solubility on the rate of anesthetic uptake. If $F_I = 0.5$ (50%), then $\lambda' = \lambda \times (1 - 0.5) = 0.5\lambda$. This is how the model needs to be adapted to account for the second gas effect of breathing 50% nitrous oxide.

What must happen to the tissue/gas partition coefficient to accurately predict the λ' to be used for tissues? If F_I is 50%, must the tissue/gas partition coefficient be decreased to half as well? My intuition is that the tissue/gas partition must change because plasma/tissue solubility should remain unchanged. However, I never got around to working this out mathematically.

A Reflection

Much of my life has focused on the factors that govern how anesthetics move within the body, movements that dictate how anesthetics act and why the actions differ among anesthetics with different solubilities. Friends and colleagues have led me in this world of pharmacokinetics: John Severinghaus, Larry Saidman, Phil Larson, Edwin Munson, Ty Smith, Bob Stoelting, Wendell Stevens, Eric Wahrenbrock, and Michael Halsey, to name a few.

In retrospect, I should elevate Ms. Minnie Moore, my geometry teacher, to the top of my list. Ms. Moore gave me the rules that govern shape and purpose. She showed how elegant understanding could be built on simple postulates. And she showed how the principles of geometry, logically constructed from postulates, were part of the core mathematics of science. Perhaps my decades of work were motivated by an effort to construct the principles of inhaled anesthetic uptake and distribution from scientifically testable hypotheses, just as Euclid had done for geometry more than two millennia ago.

References

1. Larson CP Jr, Eger EI II, Severinghaus JW. Ostwald solubility coefficients for anesthetic gases in various fluids and tissues. *Anesthesiology*. 1962;23:686-689.
2. Price HL. A dynamic concept of the distribution of thiopental in the human body. *Anesthesiology*. 1960;21:40-45.
3. Severinghaus JW. Role of lung factors. In: Papper E, Kitz R, eds. *Uptake and Distribution of Anesthetic Agents*. McGraw-Hill; 1963:59-71.
4. MacKrell TN. An electrical teaching model. In: Papper EM, Kitz RJ, eds. *Uptake and Distribution of Anesthetic Agents*. McGraw-Hill Book Company, Inc; 1963:215-223:chap 17.
5. Mapleson WW. Quantitative prediction of anesthetic concentrations. In: Papper EM, Kitz RJ, eds. *Uptake and Distribution of Anesthetic Agents*. McGraw-Hill; 1963:104-119:chap 9.
6. Perl W, Lesser GT, Steele JM. The kinetics of distribution of the fat-soluble inert gas cyclopropane in the body. *Biophys J*. 1960;1:111-135.
7. Perl W. Large-scale diffusion between body compartments. In: Papper EM, Kitz RJ, eds. *Uptake and Distribution of Anesthetic Agents*. McGraw-Hill Book Company, Inc; 1963:224-227:chap 18.
8. Eger EI II. The effect of inspired concentration on the rate of rise of alveolar concentration. *Anesthesiology*. 1963;24:153-157.
9. Eger EI II, Guadagni NP. Halothane uptake in man at constant alveolar concentration. *Anesthesiology*. 1963;24:299-304.
10. Rampil IJ, Mason P, Singh H. Anesthetic potency (MAC) is independent of forebrain structures in the rat. *Anesthesiology*. 1993;78:707-712.
11. Antognini JF, Schwartz K. Exaggerated anesthetic requirements in the preferentially anesthetized brain. *Anesthesiology*. 1993;79:1244-1249.
12. Faulconer A, Pender JW, Bickford RG. The influence of partial pressure of nitrous oxide on the depth of anesthesia and the electroencephalogram in man. *Anesthesiology*. 1949;10:601-609.
13. Faulconer A Jr. Correlation of concentrations of ether in arterial blood with electro-encephalographic patterns occurring during ether-oxygen and during nitrous oxide, oxygen and ether anesthesia of human surgical patients. *Anesthesiology*. 1952;13:361-369.
14. Eger EI II, Johnson EA, Larson CP Jr, Severinghaus JW. The uptake and distribution of intravenous ether. *Anesthesiology*. 1962;23:647-650.
15. Hull CJ, Van Beem HB, McLeod K, Sibbald A, Watson MJ. A pharmacodynamic model for pancuronium. *Br J Anaesth*. 1978;50:1113-1123.
16. Sheiner LB, Stanski DR, Vozeh S, Miller RD, Ham J. Simultaneous modeling of pharmacokinetics and pharmacodynamics: application to d-tubocurarine. *Clin Pharmacol Ther*. 1979;25:358-371.
17. Purdon PL, Sampson A, Pavone KJ, Brown EN. Clinical electroencephalography for anesthesiologists. Part I: background and basic signatures. *Anesthesiology*. 2015;123:937-960.
18. Eger EI II. Respiratory and circulatory factors in uptake and distribution of volatile anaesthetic agents. *Br J Anaesth*. 1964;36:155-171.
19. Munson ES, Eger EI II, Bowers DL. Effects of anesthetic-depressed ventilation and cardiac output on anesthetic uptake: a computer nonlinear stimulation. *Anesthesiology*. 1973;38:251-259.

20. Brandstater B, Eger EI II, Edelist G. Effects of halothane, ether and cyclopropane on respiration. *Br J Anaesth*. 1965;37:890-897.

21. Eger EI II, Smith NT, Stoelting RK, Cullen DJ, Kadis LB, Whitcher CE. Cardiovascular effects of halothane in man. *Anesthesiology*. 1970;32:396-409.

22. Eger EI II, Smith NT, Cullen DJ, Cullen BF, Gregory GA. A comparison of the cardiovascular effects of halothane, fluroxene, ether and cyclopropane in man: a resume. *Anesthesiology*. 1971;34:25-41.

23. Gibbons RT, Steffey EP, Eger EI II. The effect of spontaneous versus controlled ventilation on the rate of rise of alveolar halothane concentration in dogs. *Anesth Analg*. 1977;56:32-34.

24. Cromwell TH, Stevens WC, Eger EI II, et al. The cardiovascular effects of compound 468 (Forane) during spontaneous ventilation and CO_2 challenge in man. *Anesthesiology*. 1971;35:17-25.

25. Calverley RK, Smith NT, Jones CW, Prys-Roberts C, Eger EI II. Ventilatory and cardiovascular effects of enflurane anesthesia during spontaneous ventilation in man. *Anesth Analg*. 1978;57:610-618.

26. Calverley RK, Smith NT, Prys-Roberts C, Eger EI II, Jones CW. Cardiovascular effects of enflurane anesthesia during controlled ventilation in man. *Anesth Analg*. 1970,57.619-628.

27. Eger EI II, Dolan WM, Stevens WC, Miller RD, Way WL. Surgical stimulation antagonizes the respiratory depression produced by Forane. *Anesthesiology*. 1972;36:544-549.

28. France CJ, Plumer HM, Eger EI II, Wahrenbrock EA. Ventilatory effects of isoflurane (Forane) or halothane when combined with morphine, nitrous oxide and surgery. *Br J Anaesth*. 1974;46:117-120.

29. Eger EI II, Bahlman SH, Munson ES. The effect of age on the rate of increase of alveolar anesthetic concentration. *Anesthesiology*. 1971;35:365-372.

30. Wahrenbrock EA, Eger EI II, Laravuso RB, Maruschak G. Anesthetic uptake – of mice and men (and whales). *Anesthesiology*. 1974;40:19-23.

31. Gregory GA, Eger EI II, Munson ES. The relationship between age and halothane requirement in man. *Anesthesiology*. 1969;30:488-491.

32. Stevens WC, Dolan WM, Gibbons RT, et al. Minimum alveolar concentrations (MAC) of isoflurane with and without nitrous oxide in patients of various ages. *Anesthesiology*. 1975;42:197-200.

33. Eger EI II, Bahlman SH, Halsey MJ, Sawyer DC. The effect of distribution of increased cardiac output on the pulmonary exchange of halothane, nitrous oxide, and methoxyflurane. *Anesth Analg*. 1973;52:625-631.

34. Blaak EE, van Baak MA, Kemerink GJ, Pakbiers MT, Heidendal GA, Saris WH. Beta-adrenergic stimulation and abdominal subcutaneous fat blood flow in lean, obese, and reduced-obese subjects. *Metabolism*. 1995;44:183-187.

35. Munson ES, Eger EI II. The effects of hyperthermia and hypothermia on the rate of of induction of anesthesia: calculations using a mathematical model. *Anesthesiology*. 1970;33:515-519.

36. Eger EI II, Saidman LJ, Brandstater B. Temperature dependence of halothane and cyclopropane anesthesia in dogs: correlation with some theories of anesthetic action. *Anesthesiology*. 1965;26:764-770.

37. Eger EI II, Johnson BH. MAC of I-653 in rats, including a test of the effect of body temperature and anesthetic duration. *Anesth Analg*. 1987;66:974-976.

38. Eger EI II, Larson CP Jr. Anaesthetic solubility in blood and tissues: values and significance. *Br J Anaesth*. 1964;36:140-144.

39. Eger EI II, Babad AA, Regan MJ, Larson CP Jr, Shargel R, Severinghaus JW. Delayed approach of arterial to alveolar nitrous oxide partial pressures in dog and in man. *Anesthesiology*. 1966;27:288-297.

40. Eger EI II, Severinghaus JW. Effect of uneven pulmonary distribution of blood and gas on induction with inhalation anesthetics. *Anesthesiology*. 1964;25:620-626.

41. Stoelting RK, Longnecker DE. The effect of right-to-left shunt on the rate of increase of arterial anesthetic concentration. *Anesthesiology*. 1972;36:352-356.

42. Perl W, Rackow H, Salanitre E, Wolf GL, Epstein RM. Intertissue diffusion effect for inert fat-soluble gases. *J Appl Physiol*. 1965;20:621-627.

43. Rackow H, Salanitre E, Epstein RM, Wolf GL, Perl W. Simultaneous uptake of nitrous oxide and cyclopropane in man as a test of compartment model. *J Appl Physiol*. 1965;20:611-620.

44. Mencken HL. *Prejudices – Second Series Chapter 4: The Divine Afflatus*. Alfred A. Knopf; 1920.

45. Lockhart SH, Eger EI II. Absence of abundant saturable binding sites for halothane or isoflurane in rabbit brain: inhaled anesthetics obey Henry's law. *Anesth Analg*. 1990;71:70-72.

46. Gregory GA, Eger EI II. Inhalation anesthesia: pharmacokinetics. In: Gray TC, Nunn JF, eds. *General Anaesthesia*. Butterworths; 1971:439-464.

47. Carpenter RL, Eger EI II, Johnson BH, Unadkat JD, Sheiner LB. Pharmacokinetics of inhaled anesthetics in humans: measurements during and after the simultaneous administration of enflurane, halothane, isoflurane, methoxyflurane, and nitrous oxide. *Anesth Analg*. 1986;65:575-582.

48. Carpenter RL, Eger EI II, Johnson BH, Unadkat JD, Sheiner LB. Does the duration of anesthetic administration affect the pharmacokinetics or metabolism of inhaled anesthetics in humans. *Anesth Analg*. 1987;66:1-8.

49. Yasuda N, Targ AG, Eger EI II, Johnson BH, Weiskopf RB. Pharmacokinetics of desflurane, sevoflurane, isoflurane, and halothane in pigs. *Anesth Analg*. 1990;71:340-348.

50. Yasuda N, Lockhart SH, Eger EI II, et al. Comparison of kinetics of sevoflurane and isoflurane in humans. *Anesth Analg*. 1991;72:316-324.

51. Yasuda N, Lockhart SH, Eger EI II, et al. Kinetics of desflurane, isoflurane, and halothane in humans. *Anesthesiology*. 1991;74:489-498.

52. Strum DP, Eger EI II, Unadkat JD, Johnson BH, Carpenter RL. Age affects the pharmacokinetics of inhaled anesthetics in humans. *Anesth Analg*. 1991;73:310-318.

53. Allott PR, Steward A, Mapleson WW. Pharmacokinetics of halothane in the dog. Comparison of theory and measurement in individuals. *Br J Anaesth*. 1976;48:279-295.

54. Stoelting RK, Eger EI II. The effects of ventilation and anesthetic solubility on recovery from anesthesia: an in vivo and analog analysis before and after equilibration. *Anesthesiology*. 1969;30:290-296.

55. Eger EI II, Johnson BH. Rates of awakening from anesthesia with I-653, halothane, isoflurane, and sevoflurane: a test of the effect of anesthetic concentration and duration in rats. *Anesth Analg*. 1987;66:977-982.

56. Eger EI II, Gong D, Koblin DD, et al. Effect of anesthetic duration on kinetic and recovery characteristics of desflurane vs. sevoflurane (plus compound A) in volunteers. *Anesth Analg.* 1998;86:414-421.

57. Nordmann GR, Read JA, Sale SM, Stoddart PA, Wolf AR. Emergence and recovery in children after desflurane and isoflurane anaesthesia: effect of anaesthetic duration. *Br J Anaesth.* 2006;96:779-785.

58. McKay RE, Malhotra A, Cakmakkaya OS, Hall KT, McKay WR, Apfel CC. Effect of increased body mass index and anaesthetic duration on recovery of protective airway reflexes after sevoflurane vs desflurane. *Br J Anaesth.* 2010;104:175-182.

59. Saidman LJ, Eger EI II. The effect of thiopental metabolism on duration of anesthesia. *Anesthesiology.* 1966;27:118-126.

60. Saidman LJ, Eger EI II. Uptake and distribution of thiopental after oral, rectal, and intramuscular administration: effect of hepatic metabolism and injection site blood flow. *Clin Pharmacol Ther.* 1973;14:12-20.

61. Morio M, Fujii K, Satoh N, et al. Reaction of sevoflurane and its degradation products with soda lime. Toxicity of the byproducts. *Anesthesiology* 1992;77:1155-1164.

62. Fang ZX, Eger EI II, Laster MJ, Chortkoff BS, Kandel L, Ionescu P. Carbon monoxide production from degradation of desflurane, enflurane, isoflurane, halothane, and sevoflurane by soda lime and Baralyme. *Anesth Analg.* 1995;80:1187-1193.

63. Halsey MJ, Sawyer DC, Eger EI II, Bahlman SH, Impelman DM. Hepatic metabolism of halothane, methoxyflurane, cyclopropane, Ethrane, and Forane in miniature swine. *Anesthesiology.* 1971;35:43-47.

64. Sawyer DC, Eger EI II, Bahlman SH, Cullen BF, Impelman D. Concentration dependence of hepatic halothane metabolism. *Anesthesiology.* 1971;34:230-235.

65. Sawyer D, Eger E II. Hepatic metabolism of halothane. *Int Anesthesiol Clin.* 1974;12:55-62.

66. Hitt BA, Mazze RI, Beppu WJ, Stevens WC, Eger EI II. Enflurane metabolism in rats and man. *J Pharmacol Exp Ther.* 1977;203:193-202.

67. Cahalan MK, Johnson BH, Eger EI II, et al. A noninvasive in vivo method of assessing the kinetics of halothane metabolism in humans. *Anesthesiology.* 1982;57:298-302.

68. White AE, Stevens WC, Eger EI II, Mazze RI, Hitt BA. Enflurane and methoxyflurane metabolism at anesthetic and at subanesthetic concentrations. *Anesth Analg.* 1979;58:221-224.

69. Cahalan MK, Johnson BH, Eger EI II. Relationship of concentrations of halothane and enflurane to their metabolism and elimination in man. *Anesthesiology.* 1981;54:3-8.

70. Klan PH, Herden HN, Lawin P. Gaschromatographic examination of the expired air after anaesthesia with halothane, enflurane and methoxyflurane (author's transl). *Prakt Anaesth.* 1975;10:356-360.

71. Munson ES, Eger EI II, Tham MK, Embro WJ. Increase in anesthetic uptake, excretion, and blood solubility in man after eating. *Anesth Analg.* 1978;57:224-231.

72. Munson ES, Merrick HC. Effect of nitrous oxide on venous air embolism. *Anesthesiology.* 1966;27:783-787.

73. Eger EI II, Saidman LJ. Hazards of nitrous oxide anesthesia in bowel obstruction and pneumothorax. *Anesthesiology.* 1965;26:61-66.

74. Steffey EP, Johnson BH, Eger EI II, Howland D Jr. Nitrous oxide: effect on accumulation rate and uptake of bowel gases. *Anesth Analg.* 1979;58:405-408.

75. Steffey EP, Johnson BH, Eger EI II. Nitrous oxide intensifies the pulmonary arterial pressure response to venous injection of carbon dioxide in the dog. *Anesthesiology.* 1980;52:52-55.

76. Stanley TH, Kawamura R, Graves C. Effects of nitrous oxide on volume and pressure of endotracheal tube cuffs. *Anesthesiology.* 1974;41:256-262.

77. Lumb AB, Wrigley MW. The effect of nitrous oxide on laryngeal mask cuff pressure. In vitro and in vivo studies. *Anaesthesia.* 1992;47:320-323.

78. Kaplan R, Abramowitz MD, Epstein BS. Nitrous oxide and air-filled balloon-tipped catheters. *Anesthesiology.* 1981;55:71-73.

79. Eisenkraft JB, Eger EI II. Nitrous oxide anesthesia may double the balloon gas volume of Swan-Ganz catheters. *Mt Sinai J Med.* 1982;49:430-433.

80. Saidman LJ, Eger EI II. Change in cerebrospinal fluid pressure during pneumoencephalography under nitrous oxide anesthesia. *Anesthesiology.* 1965;26:67-72.

81. Seaberg RR, Freeman WR, Goldbaum MH, Manecke GR Jr. Permanent postoperative vision loss associated with expansion of intraocular gas in the presence of a nitrous oxide-containing anesthetic. *Anesthesiology.* 2002;97:1309-1310.

82. Artru A, Sohn YJ, Eger EI II. Increased intracranial pressure from nitrous oxide five days after pneumoencephalography. *Anesthesiology.* 1978;49:136-137.

83. Eger EI II, Ethans CT. The effects of inflow, overflow and valve placement on economy of the circle system. *Anesthesiology.* 1968;29:93-100.

84. Harper M, Eger EI II. A comparison of the efficiency of three anesthesia circle systems. *Anesth Analg.* 1976;55:724-729.

85. Stoelting RK, Eger EI II. Percutaneous loss of nitrous oxide, cyclopropane, ether and halothane in man. *Anesthesiology.* 1969;30:278-283.

86. Fassoulaki A, Lockhart SH, Freire BA, et al. Percutaneous loss of desflurane, isoflurane, and halothane in humans. *Anesthesiology.* 1991;74:479-483.

87. Lockhart SH, Yasuda N, Peterson N, et al. Comparison of percutaneous losses of sevoflurane and isoflurane in humans. *Anesth Analg.* 1991;72:212-215.

88. Cullen BF, Eger EI II. Diffusion of nitrous oxide, cyclopropane, and halothane through human skin and amniotic membrane. *Anesthesiology.* 1972;36:168-173.

89. Laster MJ, Taheri S, Eger EI II, Liu J, Rampil IJ, Dwyer R. Visceral losses of desflurane, isoflurane, and halothane in swine. *Anesth Analg.* 1991;73:209-212.

90. Merkel G, Eger EI II. A comparative study of halothane and halopropane anesthesia including method for determining equipotency. *Anesthesiology.* 1963;24:346-357.

91. Epstein RM, Rackow H, Salanitre E, Wolf GL. Influence of the concentration effect on the uptake of anesthetic mixtures: the second gas effect. *Anesthesiology.* 1964;25:364-371.

92. Stoelting RK, Eger EI II. An additional explanation for the second gas effect: a concentrating effect. *Anesthesiology.* 1969;30:273-277.

93. Taheri S, Eger EI II. A demonstration of the concentration and second gas effects in humans anesthetized with nitrous oxide and desflurane. *Anesth Analg.* 1999;89:774-780.

94. Eger EI II, Smith RA, Koblin DD. The concentration effect can be mimicked by a decrease in blood solubility. *Anesthesiology.* 1978;49:282-284.

Family 9

Moving to California

Dr. Al Rutner and his wife, Phyllis, were among our dearest friends in Fort Leavenworth. Al was another Berry Plan draftee. We overlapped for 1 year at Ft. Leavenworth before Al left for a urology residency at UCSF. Having decided to pursue my own postmilitary training at UCSF, I reached out to Al for help with the logistics of moving to San Francisco. Al found us a home to rent in Daly City. The price was right, but we didn't realize that this was the foggiest and coldest part of the city, particularly in the summer.

There is great truth to the quote, commonly (but incorrectly) attributed to Mark Twain, that "The coldest winter I ever spent was a summer in San Francisco." Arriving in Daly City in the early summer, Cris and Dori (**Figure 9.1**) were constantly bundled up in our chilly new home. Dori developed a persistent nasal discharge that we called the "green worm." It took a fall trip to Yosemite for us to finally find the sun. Adding to the stress on Dollie, she was now pregnant with our third child, Edmond I Eger III, born in January 1961. Two years later we had our fourth and final child, Renee Ross Eger.

Greenbrae

When my fellowship ended, I was offered a research position at UCSF, including a faculty salary. This allowed Dollie and me to buy a house in Greenbrae California, a city bathed in the sunshine of Marin County.

We lived in Greenbrae for nearly a quarter of a century in a conventional marriage. I was the breadwinner. Dollie raised our children (**Figures 9.1-9.3**) and conducted the household affairs. There being no education for this (still true today), we patterned our roles as adults and as parents on our observations of our own parents from our childhood. I left for work in the early morning, usually sharing a ride with colleagues. I returned for dinner, the time the entire family convened daily. The interactions at dinner differed from those I had known as a child in that our children were drawn into the conversations and pressed to describe their days' activities.

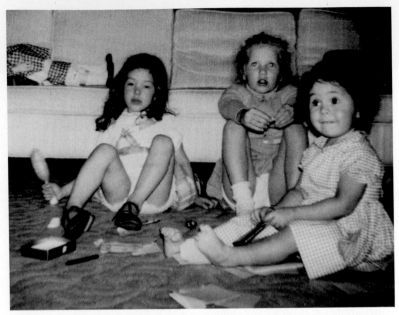

Figure 9.1 My daughter Cris Cadence (now a nurse and administrator for the emergency physicians at Bartlett Hospital in Juneau AK), cousin Kathy Jo Ogren (presently Provost of the University of Redlands), and daughter Doreen Joyce, now a practicing veterinarian, in 1961.

We reflected our upbringing in ways that occasionally surprised us. I recall one memorable evening when Dollie instructed Cris "Tell your father what you did" (an ominous beginning). Head down, Cris said that she and her friends played at the top of a nearby hill. Part of the play included pushing a large boulder to the edge of the hill. At that point, gravity took control. The boulder gathered speed, tearing through a fence at the bottom of the hill. Continuing through the yard, it passed through the fence on the other side and came to rest. The lady of the house viewed the boulder's journey through her previously fenced property from her kitchen window. This was followed by a long pause in the dinner's conversation. I asked if anyone had been hurt. On hearing that no one had, I made the mistake of laughing (uncontrollably). My mother, who thought my climbing on a greenhouse roof funny, would have been pleased that I saw the humor in my children's exploits. Dollie was not pleased. She expected discipline to be maintained.

After dinner, I would read to each child. I often put my children to bed, singing lullabies and folk songs to them. As they got older, these practices changed to the playing of games, usually board games. Including checkers.

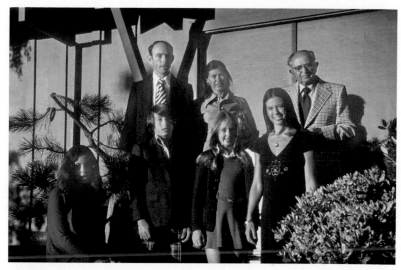

Figure 9.2 My family plus Edwin Ross, Dollie's father, early 1970s, in front of our house in Greenbrae. Front row (from left): Dori, Ed, Renee, and Cris. Back row: me, Dollie, and Ed Ross. Despite various prejudices, Ed Ross was a kind man with a sense of humor. We both liked Limburger cheese.

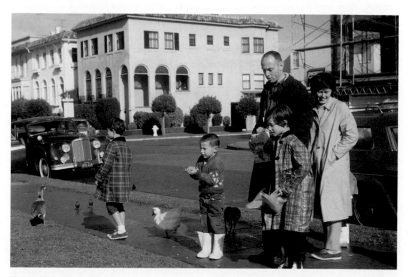

Figure 9.3 Family feeding geese and ducks mid-1960s near the Palace of Fine Arts, San Francisco (from left): Dori, Ed, me, Cris, and Dollie.

Since we had four children over the course of 6 years, the relationships among those children and their cousins probably tightened. It also provided wonderful images of uninhibited kids who perhaps now regret allowing their parents to take snapshots.

Much of my daytime life focused on my research. Our evenings offered opportunities in addition to reading to our children. Dollie was an accomplished flutist who played in amateur Marin orchestras. For a time, Renee followed her mother as a flutist, simultaneously occupying first chair in two youth orchestras. I made a halfhearted attempt to join in with a wooden flute, the recorder. Fortunately, I abandoned that effort, limiting my musical pursuits to singing. Dollie and I frequently attended performances of the San Francisco Symphony. Often, I slept through the program, but occasionally I was caught up by Seiji Ozawa's conducting a Brahms symphony. We both were attracted to plays offered by what is now the San Francisco Actor's Conservatory Theatre. These included inspiring plays like Tiny Alice by Edward Albee.

Our friends, the Rutners, drew us into another activity that was completely foreign: car camping. In later years this became back packing. The summer of our first California year we went to Yosemite Valley and opened the car door. Cris welcomed the dusty valley floor. Her pretty, clean dress soon was tinged with black, and she changed to a second clean dress. It became apparent that changing dresses was a fruitless solution, and we accepted dust as our friend. Car camping in the high Sierras developed as a summer routine for us and the Rutners. We drove to a State Park, set up our tents, and swam in the local river or lake. We would barbeque, play bridge, and chase bears away from the garbage. Who knew that barbeque in the wild could be so good and that bears were so timid?

We did other things that earlier lives had not taught us. We gathered fruits, nuts, and vegetables from Marin farms, picked berries from wild and cultivated bushes, and gathered shiny chestnuts and apples from local trees. The apples were less fun to harvest because so many could be picked so quickly. I planted my own trees, dwarf Santa Rosa plums, and conventional apricots. These produced regular harvests, which were sometimes large. Cultivating vegetables and trees gave time for quiet thinking, an activity I continued to pursue.

Our family acquired a lamb from an experiment done on a ewe with an extra lamb. Dollie was aghast, immediately assigning the lamb to my care. A wise woman. I quickly found a better home for the lamb at our local zoo. We also acquired two beagles from an experiment on dogs. Purebred beagles, Acki and Ace. Acki was so named because he had bone deformities that made him look acromegalic. A more affectionate dog could not be found. Acki stayed with us for years. Ace was too high strung for our noisy group, and like the lamb found another owner.

I Became a Professor

I developed an addiction disorder that added to our family stress. I was not addicted to drugs, except perhaps endogenous dopamine. I became addicted to research. USCF made it possible for me to not only think about how things worked, but to test my ideas in human subjects. I knew that a stay of 1 or 2 years wouldn't be sufficient to satisfy my new addiction. I wanted to join the faculty. Dr. Cullen, my guardian angel, offered me a research position at a faculty salary. He also asked me to write a review paper on atropine, scopolamine, and related compounds. I did, because I did what Dr. Cullen told me to do.[1] The review was quoted widely.

I discovered early in my career that I loved teaching residents. Teaching anesthetic pharmacology to residents sharpened my own thinking about the anesthetic uptake and distribution. In 1963, shortly after completing my own fellowship, I founded the Western Anesthesia Residents Conference (WARC). This is an annual meeting in which residents present the results of clinical or laboratory research studies. WARC has thrived and grown over the years into a vibrant annual meeting that now includes 14 academic Anesthesia Departments on the West Coast and is well attended by residents, department chairs, and anesthesia research faculty.

My work with uptake and distribution in the early 1960s made me a celebrity in my small world. Despite my junior status (a mere instructor), I was in demand for talks and visiting professorships. I was even offered positions as Director of Research at the University of Miami and the University of Washington. On the recruiting visit to Miami, I watched the locals seine for shrimp using lanterns to attract the crustaceans. Later Dollie and I looked at housing options in Southern Florida. Seeing we were serious about possibly moving, Dr. Cullen countered by making me a professor at UCSF in 1968.

We stayed, having fallen in love with San Francisco. *Besides, how could I do anything without John Severinghaus?*

Super Straight Is Coming Down

The Hubbard Street Dance Company began its life in 1974 in Chicago. I don't remember how I came to it first, but I probably saw it in one of many visits "home" to Chicago to visit friends and relatives. One of its many delights was the 1980s ballet Super Straight Is Coming Down, a wonderful comment on the chaos of modern life. I learned that Hubbard Street would be performing Super Straight at the Jacob's Pillow Dance Festival in the Birkshire Hills of Western

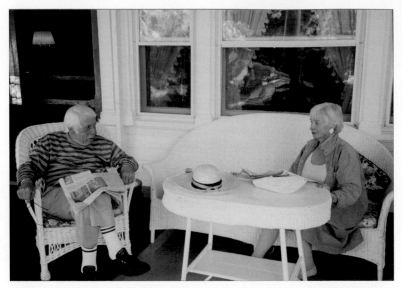

Figure 9.4   My sister, Suzanne, and her husband, Joe, on a hotel porch returning in 1990 from a performance of Super Straight is Coming Down by the Hubbard Street Dance Company at the Jacob's Pillow Dance Festival.

Massachusetts. I had been so impressed by Super Straight that when I visited my sister Suzanne and her husband Joe Roddy in nearby Croton, New York, I took them to Jacob's Pillow so they might be equally pleased (**Figure 9.4**).

Balance

My professional success coincided with unwelcome drama in my personal life. As my 50th birthday approached, I found myself married to a good woman I did not love. I don't know why this happened, other than that scientific pursuit was unexpectedly seductive and satisfying. I chose a well-established but painfully selfish solution: I opted for divorce.

I remember a few of the more painful comments Dollie made. "*We had/have a contract*" she said. She was correct. Even more painful was her statement "*I looked forward to growing old with you.*" That had been true for me, *mutatis mutandis*, but was no longer so.

In time, I found what I was seeking. However, in retrospect, I might not have chosen the same path, causing my loving and loyal wife undeserved pain. Dollie

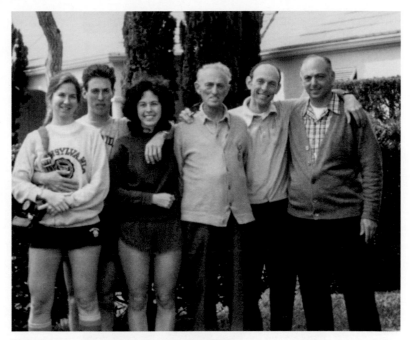

Figure 9.5   Larry's wife, Sue Burns, my half-brother, Larry, my daughter Dori, my dad, me, and my brother, Tom.

died alone, 25 years later, of colon cancer. Had we remained married, I might have guided her to a path that avoided that end. We'll never know.

Visiting Family in Sarasota

The success of the observation of MAC and its usefulness in anesthesia research and development led to many invitations to speak. Frequently these invitations took me East, and I used such opportunities to visit my father, his wife, Rebecca, and my half-brother, Larry and his family in Sarasota (**Figure 9.5**). Each trip to Sarasota followed roughly the same routine. I would eat well at my father's golf club and play one round of golf terribly with my father, achieving scores twice par at best. Despite my inept golfing, I enjoyed the opportunity to be with my father doing something he loved, something for which he had moved to Sarasota. I had the illusion that if my father and I lived long enough, his game would slowly deteriorate, eventually producing two equally inept but competitive golfers. I'd catch up with him!

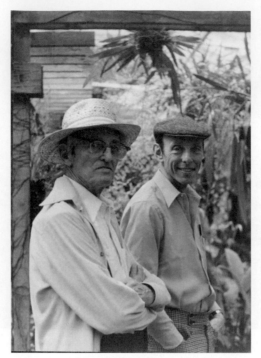

Figure 9.6   Dad and me at the Shelby Botanical Gardens.

We would have the same conversations with each visit about family history, the stock market, Rebecca's role as the Tax Collector of Sarasota County, and world affairs. I knew what each word would be, and I loved it. We would visit the Shelby Botanical Gardens (**Figure 9.6**) to see the orchids growing in rich profusion.

There was an incongruence with Rebecca's position as Sarasota County tax collector. This was particularly peculiar as this was an elected position, and Rebecca was an active Democrat in a solidly Republican county. She had been appointed to the position by a Democrat governor when the previous tax collector died. She did her job so well that when it came time for election she ran for the position and won despite her affiliation with the Democratic Party.

I particularly enjoyed my visits with my half-brother, Larry, nearly 30 years younger than I. He had grown up something of an artist-hippie. Our family despaired of what he might become. But then he decided to become a lawyer. He pursued

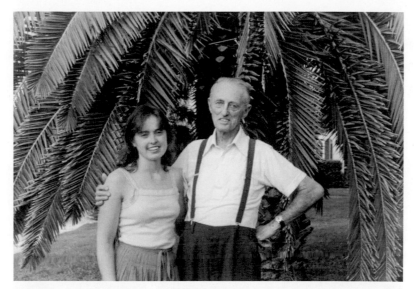

Figure 9.7   My daughter Renee and my dad, not long before his death.

a career as a public defender, eventually running for the post of Chief Public Defender. He ran as a Republican although his opponent accused him of being a RINO (Republican in Name Only). He was a relatively radical Republican.

Sarasota County thus had two elected Eger's in office: a Democratic tax collector, and a Republican public defender. It was a time when public service was defined by competence rather than political identity.

Gall Bladder Cancer

In the late 1970s, my father was diagnosed with cancer of the gall bladder that had invaded his liver. This required diversion of bile from the liver but otherwise was not an immediate threat to his life. Our family visited him more regularly (**Figure 9.7**).

Dad's cancer seemed to have little effect on his health. The diversion of bile relieved most of his symptoms. His cancer was treated with radiation. As a physician, I helped him interface with his doctors. I remember being with him while a radiologist explained the next course of treatments. Dad sat on a stool hunched forward and appeared to be falling asleep. I asked if he were all right. He said that yes, he was fine. However, if it weren't so important, he'd be bored.

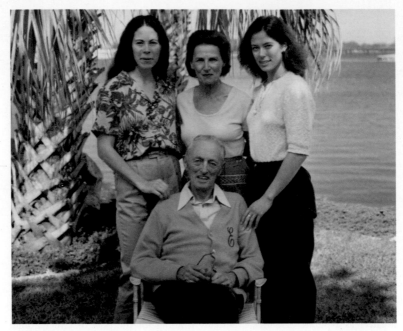

Figure 9.8 My daughter, Dori, Rebecca (dad's second wife), my daughter, Cris, and my dad.

Ever so slowly, my father slipped away. Despite the gall bladder cancer, it was his severe coronary artery disease that took his life. His angina was treated with propranolol, a beta blocker. He gradually weakened from the combination of cancer, angina, propranolol, and, perhaps, dehydration. That was followed by stupor from which he never awoke.

Figure 9.8 is one of our last family pictures with my father. He passed away on May 30, 1983.

Reference

1. Eger EI II. Atropine, scopolamine, and related compounds. *Anesthesiology*. 1962;23:365-383.

Walking in the Mountains

Meeting Tom Hornbein

John Severinghaus introduced me into the world of research, a world that became my life's work and passion. However, John was instrumental in stirring another passion: *mountains!*

In 1963, John invited me and others in the laboratory to his house to hear an anesthesiologist from the University of Washington, Dr. Thomas Hornbein, talk about his climbing Mount Everest that spring. I wasn't interested, and nearly didn't go. Who has time to climb mountains when there's so much exciting discovery about anesthesia uptake and distribution? However, John's invitation wasn't to be refused. Time was as valuable to John as it was to me. If John thought it was worth listening to Dr. Hornbein talk about climbing Mount Everest, then there must be something to it.

I listened to John's sunburnt guest, an anesthesiologist with a passion for the outdoors, describe the reasons that he climbed mountains. Dr. Hornbein told us that he wanted to find his physical and mental limits. He explained that in finding these limits, he was finding himself. The more he spoke, the more I was drawn to this philosophy. Something resonated.

I had been a weakling all my life. My lifestyle was that of a couch potato. Dr. Hornbein's talk changed that. Everest! Imagine that! As had happened so often before, John Severinghaus opened a door and, to my surprise, my life changed when I walked through.

Tom and I became good friends. He was my guide into a new world of demanding physical and mental exertion. I never became a serious mountain-eer. However, the Sierras and backpacking became part of my life. Tom included me in an expedition he organized to climb Mount Rainier. It was just half the height of Everest (14,416 ft vs 29,029 ft), but tall enough for me.

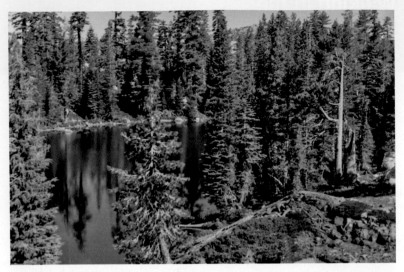

Figure 10.1   Hidden Lake.

Backpacking

Inspired by Tom, each summer from the late 1960s through the 1970s, I would take one or more of my children backpacking in the high Sierras. Sometimes I would walk with just one child as when Dori and I found Hidden Lake (**Figure 10.1**) and Lake Zitella (**Figure 10.2**), the latter a shallow high alpine lake that became warm enough in late summer to swim in comfortably. Sometimes all the children and I would walk together. Accompanied by one child or all four (**Figure 10.3**), hiking changed my life.

The John Muir Trail

In the late 1960s, two of John's fellows, Steve Bahlman and John Henry, joined me for a hike along the John Muir trail, a 211 mile footpath beginning at Happy Isles in Yosemite Valley and ending at Whitney Portal, just below Mount Whitney. At 14,505 ft, Mount Whitney was the highest summit in the contiguous United States. We divided our trip into roughly 60- to 75-mile segments. We started (and ended) each segment at a location where we could pick up food. We carried tents, sleeping and cooking gear basics, and dehydrated food. We had a grand time. Steve and John were amiable companions and able hikers (although I remember John Henry mumbling as we ascended the steepest grades: "Why me, Lord; why me?" At the end of our journey, we took the side path to the top of Mount Whitney.

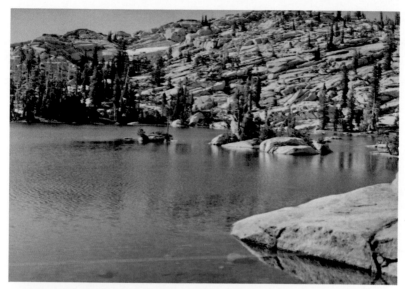

Figure 10.2 Lake Zitella.

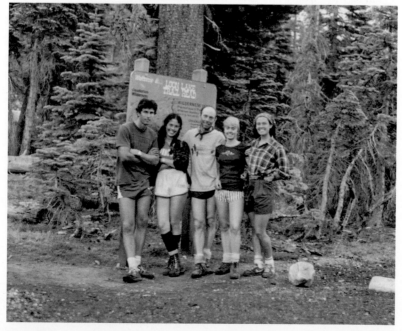

Figure 10.3 My son, Ed, daughter, Dori, me, and daughters Renee and Cris return from back-packing about 1970.

In the mid-1970s, I repeated this hike with my daughter Dori. Larry Saidman, my former fellow and then Chair of Department of Anesthesiology at the University of California at San Diego, joined us for the first portion of this adventure. While Dori and I made preparatory hikes up and down neighborhood hills, Larry attended to his chairmanly affairs in San Diego. He had little time to test the fit of his hiking boots. Larry was a bit apprehensive at our rendezvous in Yosemite Valley. On the quiet, he asked me if I thought he could keep up with me. "Sure," I said, "But I'm not the problem. Keeping up with Dori is the problem."

The first day we were scheduled to hike only 7 or 8 miles, but we hiked twice that. And the next day we also hiked much more than we had anticipated, reaching Tuolumne Meadows in record time. That sort of thing happened when Dori set the pace. Larry was a bit frazzled but game to go on. We rested that night in Tuolumne Meadows and the next day struck out for the Devil's Postpile, 30 miles away. The day was cold and windy, and clouds gradually filled the sky, pushing us to hike faster. We reached Donahue Pass at 11,000 ft and Dori and I were smiling (**Figure 10.4**). Larry was grim (**Figure 10.5**).

It began to rain, and we slogged on, up over ridges and down again into valleys filled with streams and lakes. It rained harder. We were to stop and set up camp, but we'd come so far that we hiked on, thinking of a warm motel bed at the Devil's Postpile. At one point we lost Dori who had hiked too far ahead of the old men. Frantically we pressed forward until we connected again, everyone wearing ponchos to ward off the rain. We finally reached a gravel road, perhaps 5 to 6 miles yet to go to the Devil's Postpile. We were a droopy, soggy, sad trio.

A station wagon came from behind and Larry put out his thumb. The car stopped, and we gratefully got in, sighing with relief. The occupants of the car were a grandfather and his grandson who had come to fish. Larry thanked them for picking us up and his comments became grandiloquent. He promised them they would, the next day, *catch many fish, big fish! The fish would be so big they would fill the car! There would be no room for passengers in the back! They would catch the biggest fish ever caught in the Sierras! Maybe the biggest fish in the world!* I don't know if Larry was hypoglycemic, hypotensive, or exhausted to the point of delirium, but he had obviously lost it.

Still babbling thanks, we reached the Devil's Postpile and the warmth of a motel room. Larry announced that he had developed Achilles tendonitis, and he was going to abandon this adventure. He never hiked the rest of the John Muir trail.

Larry reviewed this autobiography as I was preparing it. Time hasn't softened his memory. Larry still recalls this trip as among the worst experiences of his life.

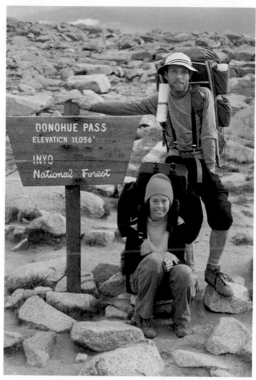

Figure 10.4   My daughter, Dori (seated), and me at Donohue Pass.

Continuing Without Larry

The remaining story comes from pleasant 50-year-old, fragmentary memories.

Dori and I resumed the trip the next morning, walking South from the Devil's Postpile, a collection of basaltic hexagonals. We adopted a routine for each day. We rose with the sun, walked an hour or two, and then stopped for a cold breakfast of Pop Tarts. We had lunch from noon to 1 PM, and then hiked on to our camp for the night near some lake or stream. When possible, we tried to end each day at low elevations where the water and air were warmer. We hung our packs from a tree to protect them from bears. We built fires from downed wood, placing our grill over the fire using flat rocks to support the grill. Each night we cooked dinner—our only hot meal for the day. Initially we walked 10 to 14 hours, covering 12 to 15 miles a day. That increased to 15 to 20 miles each day toward the end of our adventure.

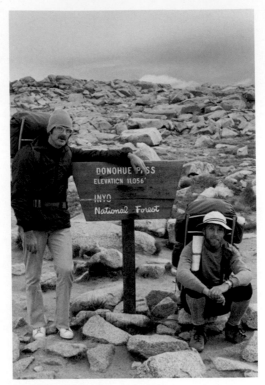

Figure 10.5   Larry (standing) and me at Donohue Pass.

On the first day, the weather was moody. It began to snow as we ascended later in the day. We didn't encounter a blizzard, but there was enough snow to cover the trail. I worried about losing the trail and getting lost. We opted for putting up the tent and holding for the night somewhere past Lake Virginia, perhaps near Silver Pass. Our stove depended on a wood fire (different from today). The weather had soaked the available wood, so we had a cold dinner.

By morning the weather had changed to clear and pleasant. It stayed that way for the remainder of our journey. Our wet clothes quickly dried.

I don't remember exactly where we stopped the second night after we left the Devil's Postpile, but I think it was near Bear Creek. We passed Marie Lake on the third day, crossing Selden Pass at just under 11,000 ft. Every day we crossed at least one pass and on a good day we would cross two. We dropped down to Heart Lake (which, of course, was shaped like a heart), and then passed between the two Sallie Keyes Lakes just below 10,000 ft. It would have been a pretty, if barren place to stop.

On day four we replenished our supplies of food, a stop we had arranged weeks before. We had plenty because we walked faster and farther than we had predicted we would each day. The pickup was just below the climb into Evolution Valley. I remember that the climb seemed steeper than the map seemed to show, perhaps because of the extra food we now carried. We stopped in Evolution Valley for the night and added wild onions to our dinner.

As we started out in the morning on the next day we met two mules amiably walking down the valley. They were followed several minutes later by a wrangler carrying halters. "They went that way" we pointed. We crossed Muir Pass at 12,000 ft where the map said, "avoid sleeping in hut" (rodents?) and continued by the Le Conte range, soon to cross Bishop Pass, also at 12,000 ft.

Much of the next day was spent between 10,000 and 13,000 ft The map showed mostly granite and little forest. We passed the Rae Lakes and ascended Glen Pass, at 13,000 ft. Hot and sweaty, we descended a bit from the pass to an unnamed pond with a small waterfowl in it. We removed our boots and waded into the cool water, pushing the waterfowl ahead of us. It was a dreadful mistake! The cooling of our muscles made it painful to then use them. Ignoring the pain, we walked on a mile or two to our night's campsite.

To the Top of Mount Whitney

The next day we walked toward Whitney Portal on a high plateau which continued for miles, and we camped two nights on this plateau.

Although the top of Mount Whitney is not a part of the John Muir trail, it is only a few miles from the trail. We couldn't resist! We deviated from the trail to ascend Mount Whitney. We reached the summit in the afternoon and decided to stay to watch the sunrise from atop this high place. As I was writing this, Dori reminded me that we found a package of Mother's Cookies at the summit. The cookies were hugely welcome, and amazing to taste. It was also amazing that the mice had left them untouched. Or, perhaps, the mice had added their own special ingredients. Maybe that says something about what's in Mother's cookies?

A hut at the top of Mount Whitney was filled with ice. We put up our tent and climbed inside to escape the cold. We awoke before light and put on all our warm clothes to watch the sun rise. A geologist joined us and told us about the origins of the rocks that surrounded us. The sun was bright but sterile. To the South we could see smog from Los Angeles streaming East.

We descended from the summit to Whitney Portal, down hundreds of traverses, dropping 7000 ft in elevation. It was afternoon by the time we reached our car and drove home. We stopped at a roadside diner. I remember ordering a steak—a tough steak laced with gristle. It was the best steak I'd ever had. Perhaps my judgment was distorted by the dehydrated food I'd been eating.

Our entire trip had taken 13 days. This hike with Dori was a special trip, one of the peak experiences of my life.

Mount Rainier

In 1970, I had tried to climb Mount Rainier with Tom Hornbein and failed. At 13,000 ft, a bit more than 1000 ft from the summit elevation, I was overcome with weariness. This was partly from inadequate training, and partly because I had reached my limits.

After many years of hiking, including my hike with Dori along the John Muir Trail described above, Tom and I talked about trying again to climb Mount Rainier. Each time I had ambivalent feelings. Yes, I wanted to expand my limits (eternal growth and youth). I remembered Tom's explanation that in finding his limits, he had found himself. However, on my first attempts to climb Mount Rainier, I had only found exhaustion and frustration. We talked more, and the negative memories faded. I again wanted to reach the top. The desire of other friends to climb Rainier and Tom's willingness to guide them created another opportunity to do so. I wanted it but my ambivalence continued to the summit.

I began training, running 3 miles daily. For the final 2 weeks of training prior to the climb I walked up stairs, 1000 ft or more each day. On Saturday, June 19, 1982, I left for Seattle. I nearly missed my flight, after locking my keys in the car on the way to the airport. A mad scramble ensued. I flagged down a van driven by an amiable elderly Black man and bribed him to drive me to my apartment and a second set of car keys. I climbed into the passenger seat of his van, finding that the seat wasn't bolted to the floor. Were the gods conspiring to kill me before I set foot on Rainier? What would Freud say?

The Party That Climbed Rainier

I arrived in Seattle and was met by Tom and Melissa, his 5-year-old daughter. Tom's wife, Kathy, joined us for a dinner of fried chicken, fruit salad, and rice on the beach of the lake their home abutted. I remember enjoying the presence of Tom, Kathy, and Melissa, and the peacefulness of that meal. We finished and turned to the business of arranging our packs. We were joined by Bill Cushman, an English teacher from Chattanooga, Tennessee. Bill was a quiet, amiable man whom I came to enjoy and respect. He had attempted to climb Rainier the previous year with Tom, but weather turned them back. Later, at bedtime, we were rewarded with hot fudge sundaes, the hot fudge being a Hornbein specialty.

We arose Sunday morning at about seven and ate a carbohydrate breakfast (croissants, rolls, and such). At nine o'clock we were met by another member of our party, Mel Stamper, a jovial 200-pound man in his late 50s who was destined to be my roommate for the next two nights. He was also the president of Boeing. I learned a bit about the 767 as the days passed. He was a gregarious presence of good will and strength.

We drove to our point of departure, stopping on the way to pick up a few last-minute supplies including a ground cover for my Steffenson-brand tent. Steffenson tents were known for their lightness and the appearance of naked ladies in their advertisements. Tom was amused at my concern for my poor tent, but he tolerated my eccentricities. At the ranger station, we completed cards attesting to our readiness (was I?) and the particulars of our route and timing. It was comforting to know that someone might come and fetch us if we didn't return. It was also distressing to think that they might need to! As mentioned above, my ambivalence persisted. We also learned that the road to the trailhead was not open. We would need to walk an additional 1.5 miles to our starting point in a campground.

We drove as far as we could, disembarked, and made final adjustments in the contents of our backpacks. Murali, a member of the Department of Anesthesia at the University of Washington, joined our party there. I received communal food and cooking gear. I suspect my pack weighed 30 to 40 lb, probably the lightest of the packs. We began our walk on a warm day. I talked with Bill Cushman about Faulkner, poets, and the process of creation. Bill was to climb Mount McKinley in the following weeks. I later learned that when he started to climb McKinley he asked himself why he was doing this. He apparently hadn't a good answer, so he turned back!

We walked in shorts and perspired. It took an hour to pass the campground and reach an inauspicious trail and the beginnings of snow, despite the warmth of the day. The trail led easily upward. I ascended it readily, my only problem being weakness of shoulders and an aching that required intermittent shifting of the pack. We reached a small stream and drank the water. Kathy worried later that it might provide giardia and diarrhea. But it was cool and tasted of dirt and salt.

We passed on to a continuous layer of snow. A stream lay under the snow. Its tributaries at times flowed under our feet. We entered Glacier Basin, a valley that led upward (like all valleys that surround Rainier). We stopped, ate, drank lemonade, and filled our bottles from the last stream we found until our descent. The trail followed the valley along its right margin for another 2 miles, reaching a steeper upward traverse called The Wedge, a narrow path leading to St. Elmo's Pass.

The Wedge led to a traverse across the south-eastern face of Burroughs Mountain. The Inter Glacier lay below. Tom, Bill, and Lynn (Tom's other daughter) led the way. I was positioned between them and Kathy and Murali. Mel was probably there as well, but I have no memory of that. The traverse to St. Elmo's Pass crossed a thirty-degree slope, down which one might slide forty feet before reaching the bottom. It was not frightening, but I wondered if I would know how to use my ice ax properly if I fell. We reached the top of the pass, which consisted of rocks and dirt. We looked down to our home for the evening, a flat space 200 ft below. I thought I had left my gloves behind but discovered after I went back to retrieve them that I had simply put them in my pocket.

I was not nearly as tired as Murali, who carried more than I despite weighing 15 lb less. At the top of the pass he sat down, saying "I'm a basket case" with both humor and seriousness.

We ambled down the steep back side of St. Elmo's Pass. The warmth of the day disappeared as the sun set and the wind rose. I had climbed in my shorts, but now put on wool knickers and wind pants, two wool sweaters, a nylon wind shirt, a down jacket, a windbreaker, and a wool hat that also served as a muffler. We carved a base for my tent and put it up with care. I instructed Mel on the "rules of the house" regarding the tenderness with which I regarded the tent. He took it all with good humor. I had positioned the tent imperfectly (I was to do that again the following night), and the wind coming across the tent caused it to cave in a bit. It flapped all night.

We attended to other tasks. A small cut in the snow served as a kitchen. Kathy was busy there with help from Tom and Lynn. Bill dug a deep ditch for sanitary purposes. He thought we had eaten more than we had, for the ditch was 2 to 3 ft deep.

Murali went to bed with a chill and then a sweat. We worried that he might have contracted a viral illness, but Kathy made the unusual diagnosis of malaria. Later we learned that he did indeed have malaria, acquired during a recent visit to Central America.

Dinner was macaroni, cheese, and tomato sauce that arrived in cans. It was the best of our meals and took a fair time to prepare. I licked the pot and felt warmed. We drank water from snow melted by our stoves, but despite that and the first of several Diamox and salt tablets, my urine was concentrated. The Diamox required an extra trip outside in the middle of a cold night wind.

We went to bed immediately after dinner. Mel quickly and easily fell asleep and snored a bit. It didn't matter; the flapping of the tent was louder than his snoring. I gradually warmed in my sleeping bag. I kept on most of my clothes but lay the down jacket under my feet. There was no headache on this or other nights. I slept well but awoke from time to time wondering if the tent fabric might tear.

We awoke Monday as we pleased, for we were waiting for Tom's son, Bob. Bob had led a party up Mount Baker and had climbed down only the night before. He had driven to the trailhead and had walked in to the campground and slept on a picnic table. He awoke early and hiked up to join us, crossing St. Elmo's Pass before 9 AM.

We had been preparing blueberry pancakes with honey or jam plus hot chocolate or other warm liquids. Murali felt better and I thought for a moment he would continue, but he was too weak. Bob quickly descended from the pass and ate the last of the blueberry pancakes. While we broke camp, Bob and Murali climbed up St. Elmo's Pass and disappeared. Bob took Murali down the steep part of the other side and returned. We learned later that Murali had had difficulty on the downhill return by himself. The fever returned, and he had to walk a hundred yards, rest, and then walk another hundred. He reached home at six that night, a longer journey than ours for that day.

We Begin the Climb

Now we roped together. Bob led Bill, Kathy, and me first on one rope. Tom took Lynn and Mel on the other. This arrangement continued for the rest of our adventure. The snow was soft from rain early in the morning, and we did not need crampons. As we advanced, the rain stopped. Bob ascended with care. We easily followed his zig-zag course among the crevasses in the surface of our glacier. We rarely retraced our steps although there were a few long traverses. I had to get used to holding the rope and adjusting its position as we moved back and forth, always keeping it downhill. I also carried an ice ax, always keeping it uphill with the point facing to the rear. That way, if I fell the point would be directed into the snow rather than into me.

We crossed blue crevasses, a few by stepping or jumping over. Others we crossed on ice-snow bridges that Bob carefully tested. The route never was steep but constantly led upward. By about 4 PM, I was pleased and surprised to see that we had reached our destination, Camp Shurman. Bill pulled me up the last 100 yards. I think he was showing off, but I didn't mind at all!

Tom and others talked to the 10 to 20 other climbers camped there. We unroped and Kathy and I focused on the outdoor john at this 10,000-foot-high place, complete with toilet paper. The rest of our group went on to our camping spot 300 to 400 ft higher. I apprehensively watched them disappear into fog. Kathy and I luxuriated in the use of the facilities and then slowly followed the group. For several hundred feet, we saw no one and I thought perhaps we would have to wait for someone to find us! But no, we topped a rise and there they were digging benches for the tents.

Mel dug one for the Steffenson tent. We knew that the tent would sit best if its back faced the wind. We put up the tent and discovered that we had misjudged the wind direction. The tent sagged where the wind blew across it and the wands supporting it twisted. Tom suggested that we reposition it and we did. The tent assumed a more "tent-like" shape but still sagged and flapped, unlike the other tents—the Early Winters Omnipotent tent and the geodesic shell, which stood shapely quiet in the breeze. I wondered what a more vigorous wind would have done to my prized Steffenson. We built short breaks on the upwind side that seemed to do little. I climbed into the tent and put on all the clothes I could find. The day was disappearing, and the air was cold and thin.

Tom and Kathy prepared dinner in the geodesic tent. It was too cold and windy to cook outside as had been done the night before. Dinner was a variant of chicken stew (cans of chicken meat). The last time I had eaten chicken stew at this altitude I had become nauseated and had not been able to face chicken in any form for months. I ate my share (no seconds) and, as anticipated, promptly felt nauseated. The nausea was probably mostly in my head, not my stomach, but I would have been wiser to stick to breakfast food. The nausea persisted all night or what there was to be of it. I have forgotten what the dessert was, but I think I forced down some hot water (I knew I had to stay hydrated or all was lost) and salt and some gorp (hiking slang for "good old raisins 'n peanuts"). And a Diamox pill.

We prepared for an early start the next day. We put our clothes in order. The rope was laid on the ground in proper lengths. Bob secured it by pressing segments into the snow (later to freeze in place). We stood outside urinating before climbing into our sleeping bags and wondering at our view of Seattle 70 miles away. I thought that the Seattleites must be warmer than we were.

Tom said we would leave at 1 AM so I set my alarm for 1 AM. Mel snored, the tent flapped, and I lay awake and worried. About what? I didn't fear falling or dying or injury of any sort except that of the soul. I feared I could not make the climb. I slept fitfully.

The alarm went off—1 AM and still dark. No one moved except Mel who awakened and asked what time it was. When I responded he asked if anyone else was up. After my "No," he allowed that he would wait until there was further activity. He soon fell asleep again. I believe he could have slept anywhere. I slowly put on the clothes I thought I would need. It seemed strange to put on suntan lotion in the darkness of the tent. Other climbers were up with lights on their heads, human Christmas brightness on a Christmas mountain. They slowly moved upwards. I struggled out of the tent, urinated, and looked at the glow of Seattle.

Tom Provides a Lift

Others awoke, dressed, and our camp slowly came to life. Kathy and Tom heated water. I drank hot water (that tasted moldy—I think from my sunburnt tongue) and forced down a mouthful of gorp. It didn't come back but another mouthful would court disaster. I asked if I might climb into the "cooking" tent for a moment of warmth and room was made.

I voiced my concern about my nausea and "maybe I shouldn't try the climb." Tom evenly suggested that a Diamox might be just the thing. He couldn't explain why but said that it worked. So, I took one and soon felt better. I collected my gear, put on my crampons, tried to attach my belt-harness. The harness didn't work so a sling-belt was made. Soon I was connected to the rope: behind Bill and ahead of Kathy, with Bob leading us all. The rope had frozen in place, and we had to work it out before we could move. It was 3:30 or 4 AM when we set out. I was bound for the summit.

Tom (**Figure 10.6**) and Bob are a large part of why I reached the top. Bob set the pace. He never hurried, and he never pushed. At the pace Bob set, there was no excuse not to keep going. We began with light the night provided: stars and the luminescence of the snow, some magical hidden fire. I do not remember being cold except for my hands from time to time. We started heading straight for the top which didn't seem that far away. However, the summit kept receding as we climbed. We avoided the crevasses and traversed back and forth, edging to the left until we crossed into another channel upwards. We had climbed an hour and a half and it seemed too easy, in part because I had started without a pack. At some point, I took my turn and shouldered the load Bob was carrying for me. My effort increased noticeably.

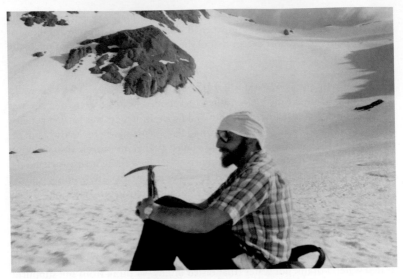

Figure 10.6　Tom Hornbein on Mount Rainier.

I ate hard candies when my aches or fatigue needed a remedy. They made my mouth moist. A crampon came loose. I sat down while Tom came up and strapped it tighter. I felt like a boy getting his shoes tied by his mommy.

Bob kicked steps into the snow frozen by the night's cold. It eased the climb both because of the improved footing and because it slowed the pace. I shifted the pack from shoulder to shoulder and from shoulders to hips and trudged on. The light increased on this, the day after the longest day of the year.

Bob pointed to a ridge, our goal in 45 minutes. He would have been there in that time had he walked alone. But it took us 2 hours. We passed another group, one near us that had lit the night at 1 AM. The group berated some poor soul named Stuart for not moving or not moving fast enough.

We reached the ridge and sat down, a sense of weariness for me. We ate carbohydrates and liquid. My lips and tongue resented the acidity of lemonade or even Gatorade. I ate snow which tasted moldy, but the fluid helped. I could have sat another hour, but Tom knew that the day wasn't going to be long enough. We set out again, spirits and strength renewed. Now we moved to the left, avoiding, I believe, an impassible crevasse. Our route took us around the mountain, to new views. How could we move around such an enormous creation in so little time? It would not have been so easy had we been at the base. Mount Hood came in view 50 miles to the South. I had but to reach through the air to touch it! Looking over its shoulder was Mount Jefferson yet another 75 miles away. We arrived at our bridge, an insubstantial crossing to the last significant part of our climb. Someone paid the troll (yes, troll) and we passed without incident.

We Reach the Top

The rim of the crater lay only a few hundred feet above us. It was late morning. Where did the time go? I was weary. I had kept the nausea at arm's length by Diamox and hard candy, but it now returned. We trudged upwards. I thought "I will get to the top, but will I have the strength to return?" The rim of the crater was barren. We crossed mud and rocks without removing our crampons. Wind blew cold and sharp across our faces.

This side of the rim was not the top. To reach that goal required us to descend into the crater and cross to the other side for a final, short, ascent. The flat floor of the crater was the size of a couple of football fields. We easily crossed its cover of firm snow, stopping at the opposite edge and unroping. I sat down, wondering where I was going to find the energy to move again while the others walked to the highest point (officially I had reached the top by crossing the rim). Kathy and Tom cajoled me into rising once more to join the group for the last few steps. I'm glad they did. At the top (Columbia Crest) we took pictures (**Figures 10.7** and **10.8**). The figure above suggests a happy but drained little boy.

The official register was kept in a sheltered place a hundred feet below the top. Each of us signed it, certifying we had come. Some noted that they had made it on the first try. I was happy to have made it at all!

The Return

Below the rim at the crater's edge we sat on brown flakey rocks, some of which were moist with steam that smelled of sulfur. We had a lunch of pilot biscuits, cheese, and sausage. Chocolate was offered, and I had some. I ate the chocolate heart that Dori had given me, and her love warmed me. We drank lemonade (or was it Gatorade? The latter seemed to go down better). The nausea subsided with the sitting. The food and liquid revived me. I had no desire to move. The sun was warm, but we could not linger.

We arose and joined together with ropes. Kathy led our group now, back across the snowy crater, up the opposite rim, across the rocky edge, and out onto the sloping snowy icy shoulder of the mountain. We retraced our steps, moving faster in descent, but careful not to move too fast and lose control.

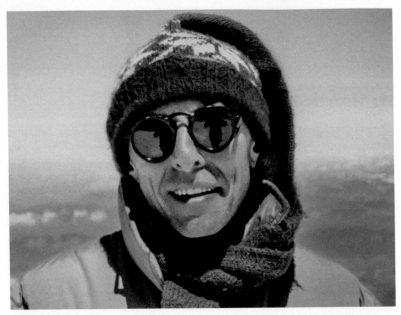

Figure 10.7   Me at the top of Mount Rainier.

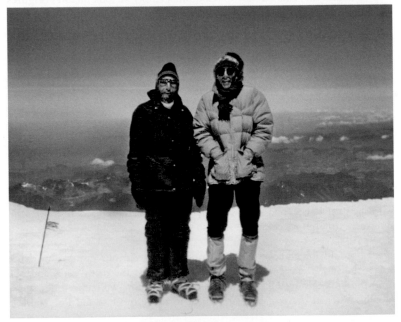

Figure 10.8   Tom and me at the top of Mount Rainier.

I was instructed in the art of self-arrest, and I had practiced it in my mind. Fortunately, I didn't need to draw upon this new-old knowledge.

We found the bridge and carefully crossed, now traversing around the shoulder, keeping high to avoid taking a false route. We found the ridge at which we had stopped to rest after passing Stuart's party. We plodded on. Our tents were in view; tiny distant colored boxes, yet another hour away.

The character of the snow changed as we descended—hard at the top but softer lower down in the afternoon sun. Sometimes it gave way and I would sink down a foot. How wasteful to lift my foot out of one hole only to move downward again in the next hole. We took a wrong turn and discovered that the "trail" led to a crevasse. We back-tracked and went around to another chute. We made the first of our glissades: we sat down, one behind the other, and the first person would slide down the snow on his/her behind. When the rope played out the next would follow and then the next. Children on a slide with a lot of laughter. Snow caught in my crotch and slowed me down. I tried to scoop it out and lost control in the process. Although the glissade sped our descent, it required more energy.

We reached the tents and set about taking them down and repacking our backpacks. I had orthostatic hypotension, probably from dehydration. I drank lemonade and ate some salt. The hypotension decreased dramatically.

We continued our descent, passing Camp Shurman. I looked longingly at the outdoor john. We went to the right and crossed a ridge to the Inter Glacier. Where to cross? Bob advocated a direct approach which might avoid some crevasses and Tom argued for a longer route that required less ascent. We ascended to the top of the ridge and walked onto the glacier. Then a series of glissades quickly brought us down 3000 ft. Several times I sped out of control, swaying like an ungainly inner tube. Snow came from everywhere. About half way down we unroped, and we slid down independently. The last one to slide went fastest because the ones before had smoothed the track. At the end, I had a wet backside and a hole in my pants.

The slope became too gentle to permit sliding, so we shouldered our packs and walked down. By now it was 7 or 8 PM, but still light. The walking became easier at the lower altitudes, but I noticed that the glissades had deposited water in my boots, and each step had a slosh to it. The boots took days to dry out, and before they did they became moldy.

We separated into groups of two or three and talked as we descended. The pace was neither leisurely (darkness would soon come) nor rapid (we were too tired for that). Groups separated, came together, changed partners, and went on, a loosely articulated single being. Conversation increased as the effort of our steps and the altitude decreased. Water flowed under the snow and Mel fell through into a streamlet. There are advantages to lightness. Snow gave way to patches of dirt, the dirt became dominant, and an undulating trail appeared. We met rangers setting out and they told us that we still had a mile and a half to go before we reached the campground. And another mile plus to reach the car. They also told us that Murali had come down safely. My shoulders ached, and I shifted the pack from shoulder to shoulder and from shoulders to hips but nothing gave more than momentary comfort. My calves ached and complained even more the next day. I did no stair climbing that day, and Kathy and I talked about the parasitic disease that we might have ingested in our drinking stream water.

Withal the last part of the day was a good time. The sun disappeared and just before darkness overtook us, we reached the campground we had left 2 days earlier. The trail became a road whose edges could be seen, even in the gloom of the late evening. Kathy and I commiserated, discussed parasites again, life (a good juxtaposition), people, and the virtues of psychoanalysis.

The cars came into view. Cars never looked so inviting! The packs came off our backs. We exchanged our boots for dry socks and our shoes for sandals. We paired into our cars. I joined Mel and Kathy for the drive to Seattle. At the ranger station at the entrance to the park we reported that we had come down safely. It was 11 PM when we set off for Seattle. I tried to stay awake and talk with Mel so that he would not doze at the wheel. I was only modestly successful. Mel got sleepy and turned the controls over to his copilot, Kathy.

It took 2 hours to reach the Hornbein's home in Seattle. I drank fruit juices while unpacking-repacking. My tongue and burnt lips resented the juice. The lips later peeled several times. My mouth felt stale, supplemented with a taste of moldy sulfur. Kathy suggested that was a sign of the parasitic infestation we had discussed. I showered and went to bed.

Sleep was short. I was up at 6:10 and by 6:30 was in a cab to the airport. I arrived none too soon. The airport was jammed, and I was nearly the last one on the plane. We flew into a clear sky, and I got another picture of Mount Rainier.

I had finished my journey.

Mount Kinabalu

The Sierra mountains had taken me to a world of wonders and pleasures. We had put our shelter, food, cooking gear, and clothing on our backs and spent days backpacking. Sometimes it led further afield, as in the climb of Mount Rainer.

My son, Ed, worked in Singapore in 1995. He invited me to climb Mount Kinabalu, at 13,438 ft, the tallest mountain in Malaysia. And so we did, in great style! Mount Kinabalu had an elegant lodge, Laban Rata Rest House, at 10,735 ft. We nearly didn't make the trip: our plane to Borneo lost the use of an engine on the way there.

We hiked a well-maintained trail up to Laban Rata, admiring orchids and pitcher plants along the way. Workers carrying supplies to the lodge strode past us, walking much faster despite carrying heavy loads. Women passed us carrying propane tanks on their backs. The tanks were held in place with a strip of tree bark around their foreheads.

We stayed the evening at Laban Rata. The next morning, we hiked to the peak before the sun rose. An unexpected bonus was to meet Chris Halsey, the daughter of a colleague and dear friend, Michael Halsey. By coincidence she had climbed Kinabalu at the same time we did, and also stayed in Laban Rata. She was as surprised to see us as we to see her.

Walking in the mountains brought joy to my life, made me healthier and happier, and allowed me to enjoy some wonderful, memorable times with my children and my friends. It also led to the next chapter in my life. I met and married a wonderful woman who enjoyed hiking, backpacking, and bird-watching. She wouldn't have been interested in me if I had remained the couch potato I had previously been.

> ### *PROMISES*
> #### *Written for our wedding*
> *We come today with promises in our pockets,*
> *Large words like always and forever,*
> *Difficult to grasp, like tumbling rockets.*
> *For the sun does not always shine or the birds sing,*
> *And though always and forever surround this ring,*
> *Better that I give you the everyday thing.*
> *I promise always perfect weather*
> *On roads we walk alone together.*
> *I'll hold your hand and cross the street.*
> *At night I'll lift and rub your feet.*
> *Evenings I shall set the table and*
> *While passing from napkins to knives,*
> *I shall catch you round the waist*
> *As husbands will with wives.*
> *And later, when dark has come,*
> *Except for reflections of the sun,*
> *I shall gather the evening tea*
> *And turn on lights for poetry.*
>
> *—Ted 1996*

Lynn

My personal life changed in the 1990s. I fell in love again! After several years of friendship blossoming into love, in 1996, I married Dr. Lynn Spitler (**Figure 11.1**). Lynn is a world-class immunologist who is primarily interested in the care of patients with melanoma. She believed in the importance of the immune system to the management of cancer decades before that importance was proven. Lynn shares my passion for walking in the mountains; indeed, she said she wouldn't have been interested in me if I had remained the couch potato I was before Tom Hornbein changed all that. I find honesty compelling, both in research partners and in life partners. Now, even after 21 years of marriage, Lynn's honesty makes me smile. Early in our relationship, I had season tickets

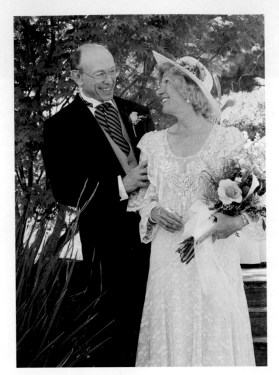

Figure 11.1   My wedding to Lynn in 1996.

to the symphony. I asked her to a performance. *"No thank you; I don't go to the symphony. I'm not interested"* she responded. I abandoned my subscription.

Our family grew with this marriage. Lynn brought her daughter, Diane Anderson, and son, Paul Spitler, into the family. All our children married and had children (totaling, for our combined families, 6 children, 6 spouses of children, and 14 grandchildren). They shared my passion for walking in the mountains, and we had many backpacking trips in the Sierras. They also joined us in Mendocino.

Mendocino is a special place for me. Lynn and I stay at the Headlands House at the edge of town, overlooking the ocean. *There my heart sings!* We walk through Headlands State Park (**Figure 11.2**) and hike the trails to Fern Canyon. We often have dinner at the picturesque Ledford House, right on the water in Albion. I often ask the instrumentalist to play "Our Love is Here to Stay." Sentimental Ted!

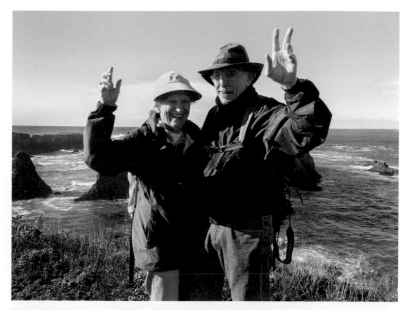

Figure 11.2   Lynn and me hiking in Mendocino Headlands State Park.

Lynn's favorite is the Kihei coast of Maui (**Figure 11.3**). We usually walk hand in hand along the beach during the day and dine on fish and seaweed at night. Lynn snorkels. I watch (more on this below).

Whenever possible, we invite our children and friends to accompany us on our trips to Mendocino and Hawaii.

Traveling With Lynn

Lynn and I share many passions, including dance, theater, and cross-country skiing (**Figure 11.4**). Lynn also has a passion for traveling the world, which I don't share. When I was invited to be a guest speaker in Guangzhou, China, I asked her if we should go. She thoughtfully told me to do whatever I wanted to do. When I told her I declined the invitation, she asked *"What?"* We went, of course. With Lynn as my traveling companion, the trip provided another adventure. As a bonus, we took a cruise past the karst limestone formations on the nearby Li River (**Figure 11.5**).

In 1997, Lynn took me to a meeting in Sydney, Australia, where she was an invited speaker. We went on to Heron Island, part of the Great Barrier Reef.

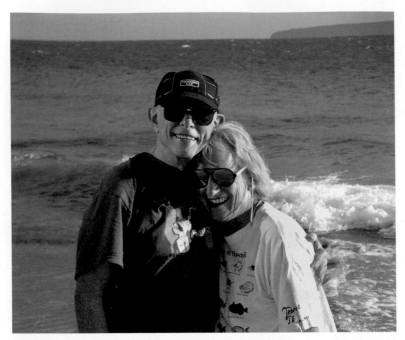

Figure 11.3 Lynn and me on the beach in Hawaii.

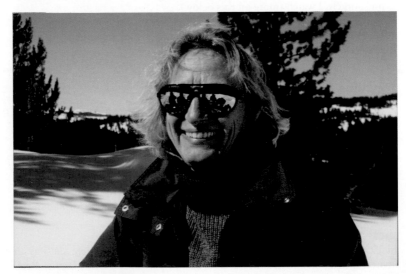

Figure 11.4 Lynn, cross-country skiing.

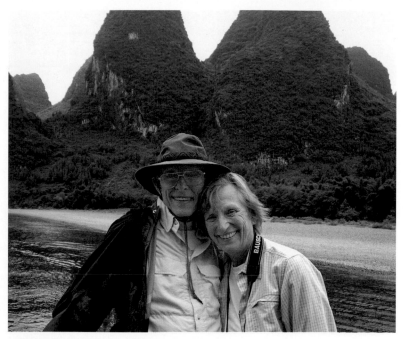

Figure 11.5   Lynn and me in China on a trip on the Li River past the karsts.

One reaches the reef by helicopter or boat. I chose boat, not wishing to fall from the sky. This may not have been the best choice. The boat ride was rough, and I became terribly seasick.

I had not snorkeled before. Lynn introduced me to the unnatural act of breathing with one's face in the water. I managed as best I could while we swam across the corals amid colorful fish. Finding shallow water, I stood up and took off my mask. Lynn asked if we were having fun. I answered, "*Yes, if being terrified is fun.*" Timid Ted!

My fear of seasickness overcame my fear of falling from the sky. The remote chance of the helicopter crashing seemed a better bet than high probability of repeating the nausea that accompanied my trip to the island. We returned by helicopter.

We visited the Blue Mountains outside of Sydney. The forest is populated by eucalyptus trees, parrots, and easy places for walking. Lynn struck up a conversation with a wallaby in a parking lot (**Figure 11.6**).

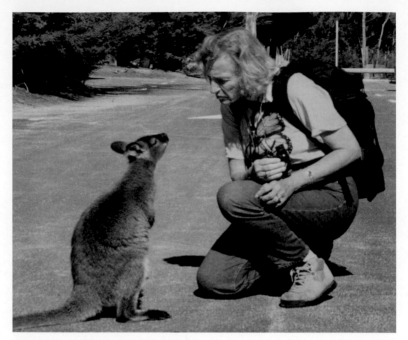

Figure 11.6   Lynn speaks with a friendly wallaby.

Painting With Lynn

I have always enjoyed painting pictures. Lynn found she also liked creating paintings. We began taking art lessons at our local Community Center, the Ranch, and continued these weekly classes for years. The teacher, Graciela, would select a picture for us to paint and show us how to paint it. We finished each painting in one or two of the weekly sessions. They are proudly on display in our garage. Special guests receive personal presentations from the artists themselves (**Figure 11.7**).

I Turn 75

I reached my 75th year in 2005. To celebrate, Lynn invited my entire family—25 of us at that time (**Figure 11.8**)—to walk 60 miles of the Pacific Crest Trail. Part of the group (including Lynn and me) started at Devil's Postpile. More joined us at Lee Vining. Before departure from Lee Vining, we enjoyed a divine dinner at a Mobile Gas Station, a restaurant now called the Whoa Nellie Deli. From there we hiked to Happy Isles in Yosemite Valley, where we were met by the rest of our party.

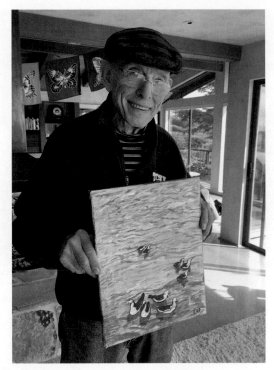

Figure 11.7 Yet another masterpiece, on loan from our garage.

This was "elegant backpacking." Horses and packers carried the food, supplies, equipment, and the necessities for shelter. It was my last major foray into the Sierras. My daughter put together a book called "Ted's 75th Birthday Camp Songs," which we enjoyed around the campfire in the evening.

We reached Half Dome on the penultimate day of our journey. Most of the family made the ascent, swallowing their terror, and determined not to let it control their lives (**Figure 11.9**). I shared their fears. I don't know if courage, foolishness, or vanity forced me to press on. However, I don't think the reason is any of these. I think it is my fatalistic view of the act, a determination to press on regardless of the cost. I have seen that in others. I saw that in Tom Hornbein, who pressed on with Willi Unsoeld over the West Ridge of Everest into an unknown night of great risk. There was no rational reason to take this risk, yet they did. Success in the face of shared risk creates bonds.

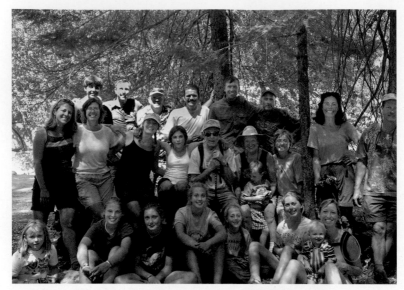

Figure 11.8   End of the family hike off the Pacific Crest Trail celebrating my 75th birthday. Front row: Ashley, Julia, Emily, Jessica, Nic, and Hannah, Leah, Ryan, Diane. Second row: Holly, Cris, Shawnee, Katharine, me, Lynn, Spencer, and Renee. Back row: William, Ed, Warren, Jamie, Paul, Steve, Dori, and Craig.

This trip was a unique and special event to share with my family. We topped it off with a hot fudge sundae brought in by our guides (**Figure 11.10**).

Merged Families

The merger of our families resulted in the development of new family traditions. One of these was a family gathering every 2 to 3 years. Everyone attended. We had family gatherings in Kings Canyon National Park in California and another in Hawaii.

Another tradition was sharing Thanksgiving with family (**Figure 11.11**). These included joining our daughter Renee and her family in Sharon, Massachusetts, which alternated with our sharing Thanksgiving with Lynn's family in Grand Rapids, Michigan.

Despite (or, perhaps, on account of) my Jewish heritage, one of our other family traditions was a lobster dinner on New Year's Eve. We usually shared this with our daughter Dori, her husband, Craig, and their son, Nic (**Figure 11.12**).

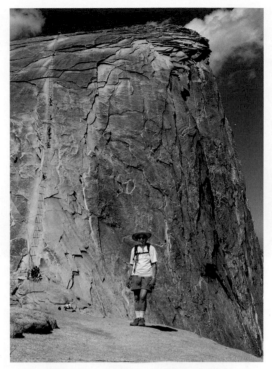

Figure 11.9 Lynn at the base of the ladder (to her left) leading to the top of Half Dome.

We brought the entire family together in 2016 to celebrate News Year's in Roatán, an island near Honduras. Our entire family came: Lynn and me, our 6 children and their spouses, all 14 grandchildren, and 2 significant others of our grandchildren. Thirty in all (**Figure 11.13**)!

These, and other, family interactions were warm, satisfying, and have added immensely to the richness of my life.

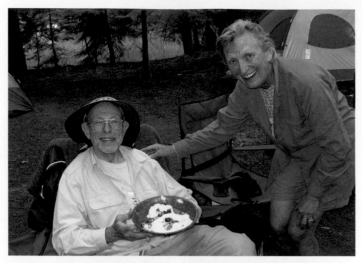

Figure 11.10 A hot fudge sundae, complete with cherry, to celebrate the evening meal on our penultimate day on the Pacific Crest trail.

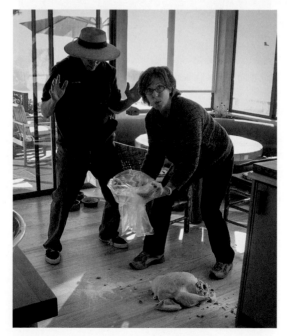

Figure 11.11 Turkeys are surprisingly slippery.

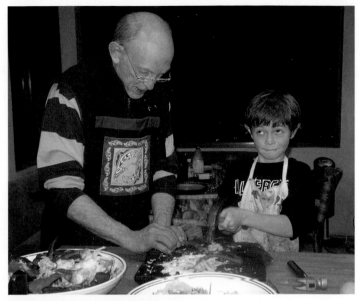

Figure 11.12 Nic and me preparing lobster on New Year's Eve.

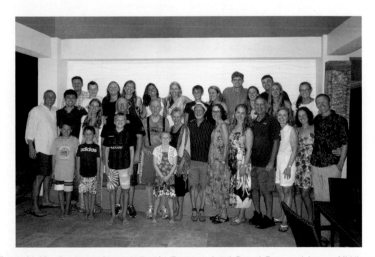

Figure 11.13 Family and friends in Roatán. Front row: Ansel, Pascal, Ryan, and Jensen. Middle row: Ed, William, Maren, Warren, me, Lynn, Craig, Don, Leah, Steve, Renee, Shawnee, and Paul. Back row: Jamie, Spencer, Ashley, Diane, Katharine, Julia, Nic, Holly, Andrew, Hannah, George, Jessica, and Cris.

Figure 11.12

Figure 11.13

New Inhaled Anesthetics

12

The Development of Modern Inhaled Anesthetics

My anesthetic career began in 1952, between my first and second years of medical school. This coincided with the introduction of the first modern inhaled anesthetics (those halogenated with fluorine). The earliest of these was fluroxene, an ethyl vinyl ether released for use in 1953. The primary advantage of fluroxene was that it didn't explode, a considerable clinical advantage over the earlier anesthetics with the potential to blow up the operating room. Fluroxene was eclipsed in the mid-1950s by halothane, an ethane synthesized by Suckling for Imperial Chemical Industries (later renamed ICI). Suckling only made 12 target compounds. By pharmaceutical standards, Suckling was either very clever or very lucky to find a blockbuster new drug from just 12 targets. Most such discoveries require synthesis of a thousand or more compounds!

I first saw halothane when it was introduced at the University of Iowa during my residency (1956-1958) for a clinical trial. The clinical benefits over fluroxene and ether were immediately obvious: halothane was highly potent (MAC = 0.75%), nonpungent, and had more rapid pharmacokinetics because of its lower solubility. Halothane quickly displaced ether at Iowa (and worldwide). In the following decades, halothane became the anesthetic against which every subsequent new anesthetic was to be compared. Halothane was also the exemplar anesthetic for studies of cardiovascular, respiratory, and other basic physiological effects of volatile anesthetics.

As mentioned in Chapter 7, halothane and I became fast friends. Halothane was the anesthetic against which I tested my theories of anesthetic potency, solubility, and the physiology responsible for anesthetic uptake and distribution. Halothane participated in my discovery of MAC, a fundamental property of inhaled anesthetics. Nearly all of what I know about inhaled anesthetics I learned from halothane.

The commercial success of halothane prompted competition for even better inhaled anesthetics. The first candidate was methoxyflurane, introduced in the early 1960s. Methoxyflurane never gained popularity because it was quickly demonstrated that it could injure the kidney. Additionally, the kinetic properties

145

of methoxyflurane were slower than halothane, and the slower uptake and distribution was not acceptable to clinicians who had become accustomed to the rapid onset and offset of halothane.

However, evidence was also emerging that halothane had rare but potentially life-threatening toxicities. In one of our early clinical studies of MAC,[1] one patient turned yellow a few days after the study. The clinical picture was acute hepatitis. However, there was no reason for this patient to develop acute hepatitis. We speculated on whether halothane might occasionally cause acute liver injury. Similar observations were being made by other clinicians, and occasionally the patients died from fulminant hepatitis after receiving halothane. The common thread was that the patients had always had a previous anesthetic with halothane. This suggested an immune mechanism, with the patient initially developing an immunological response to halothane. In such patients, a subsequent exposure triggered an immunologically mediated hepatotoxicity. As the evidence for "halothane hepatitis" became incontrovertible, a race was on to find something that retained halothane's desirable pharmacokinetics, but without the hepatotoxicity.

The Development of Isoflurane

Ohio Medical Products (OMP) was one of several companies competing to find a replacement for halothane. OMP introduced one of the first fluorinated hydrocarbons, fluoroxene, in 1951. Fluoroxene failed commercially, being somewhat flammable, but the company maintained an interest in the field. In the 1960s OMP had hired Jim Vitcha to lead their anesthetic research program. His goal was developing a new inhaled anesthetic, one that would be better and safer than the then dominant halothane. Maybe Jim had followed my short career or maybe he had asked for a recommendation for someone young and knowledgeable about inhaled anesthetics. I never knew. For whatever reason, he approached me, asking if I would like to advise Ohio Chemical Co. in its task. I didn't realize that he was asking me to be their de facto Medical Director. I said yes, beginning a half-century relationship that drew me into adventures and opportunities I never would otherwise have had.

Jim had the good sense to hire a brilliant and unassuming young fluorine chemist, Ross Terrell, to find a drug that met the high standards set by halothane, but without hepatotoxicity. Ross genius was figuring out how to synthesize peculiar fluorinated compounds. Ross synthesized more than 700 novel compounds in his search for a replacement for halothane.[2] The first of these to advance beyond laboratory trials was enflurane, an ethyl methyl ether. Enflurane was approved by the FDA in 1972, just as we were completing our basic work into the uptake, distribution, and biological effects of inhaled anesthetics.

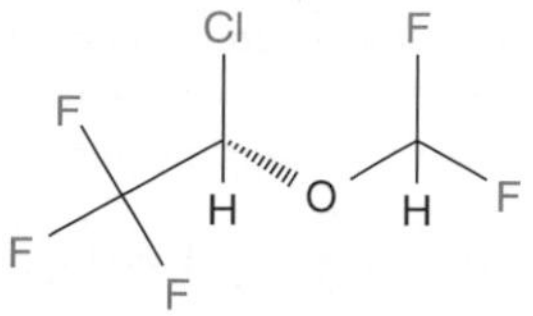

Figure 12.1   1-chloro-2,2,2-trifluoroethyl difluoromethyl ether (isoflurane).

I joined others in evaluating the anesthetics Ross made. My colleagues and I arrived too late to make a significant contribution to the study of enflurane. However, Ross had started working on another molecule, 1-chloro-2,2,2-trifluoroethyl difluoromethyl ether (**Figure 12.1**). This molecule would eventually become known to the anesthesia community as isoflurane.

Ross and his colleagues turned to our laboratory at UCSF to study isoflurane to characterize the potency, solubility, and the rates of uptake and distribution that we had defined for halothane and methoxyflurane. I was thrilled! There had been three reasons I had developed these concepts early in my career. One was that John Severinghaus had posed tough questions, and I needed the mathematics to answer them. A second reason was to guide clinical care. I knew that a patient's life hung in the balance, based on the clinician's skill with anesthetic drug administration. Knowledge was power in the hands of the anesthesiologist. My third reason was that I wanted to apply these concepts to develop the next generation of anesthetic drugs. Ross gave me that chance.

We defined many of the properties of isoflurane in humans, including isoflurane's potency (MAC),[3] and its cardiovascular,[4,5] respiratory,[6-9] electroencephalographic,[10] and neuromuscular[11] effects, including the capacity of isoflurane to augment the paralysis produced by neuromuscular blocking drugs.[12,13] Comparing isoflurane and halothane in humans, we found that isoflurane had advantageous effects on postanesthetic mentation.[14] Unlike halothane, isoflurane did not predispose to ventricular arrhythmias.[15] We showed that isoflurane had more desirable kinetic characteristics, and that the liver of swine minimally metabolized isoflurane.[16] We found little or no toxicity in humans anesthetized with isoflurane versus other inhaled anesthetics for several hours, including hours at deeper levels of anesthesia.[17]

Isoflurane demonstrated remarkable chemical stability, with virtually no evidence of metabolism. It had become clear that a trifluoroacetate metabolite mediated halothane's hepatotoxic effect. Given this, isoflurane's resistance to metabolism seemed particularly advantageous.

Our repertoire of clinical assessments grew, reflecting the expanding scope of anesthesia practice. We studied the effects of isoflurane on uterine tone, demonstrating that it increased uterine bleeding during abortions.[18] In vitro tests of *Staphylococcus aureus* demonstrated that modern potent inhaled anesthetics (including isoflurane and halothane) were lethal to *S aureus* at test vapor pressures that exceeded 35 times MAC.[19] At least some bacterial pathogens were unlikely to survive in a vaporizer charged with liquid isoflurane.

Tom Corbett's Surprise

Our extensive studies with isoflurane provided the data we anticipated that the FDA would require for clinical approval. Ohio Chemical Products prepared to submit their completed new drug application to the FDA. However, as they were preparing their application (mid-1970s) an anesthesiologist at the University of Michigan, Tom Corbett, phoned me. Tom had found evidence for carcinogenicity in fetuses exposed to isoflurane in utero and allowed to grow to late adulthood.[20] This was an unexpected finding, and a potential showstopper for isoflurane. Corbett's study had limitations in the adequacy of the controls and comparator anesthetics used. Nevertheless, a suspicion of cancer is such a devastating accusation that I believed the FDA would not approve isoflurane if it posed a risk of carcinogenesis. There was little likelihood that the FDA would dismiss findings of carcinogenesis based on arguments that the study was flawed.

I was also sure that my friends at OMP would hope that the FDA would reject Corbett's study because of the flaws in study design and execution. To me that was a nonstrategy—do nothing and hope that everything works out OK. In my view, the likely outcome was that the FDA would require OMP to repeat Corbett's study with adequate controls and comparator anesthetics. The result would be a delay of at least a year in the approval of isoflurane. Without telling either the FDA or my friends at OMP, Wendell Stevens and I set out to repeat the study on our own. Tom shared our concerns and collaborated with our efforts to repeat his work.

As predicted, isoflurane approval was blocked by the concerns about carcinogenesis. It took nearly a year for OMP to decide to ask us to repeat Tom Corbett's study. Fortunately, by the time they asked for our help, our study involving thousands of mice was well underway.

We proposed to OMP a protocol to repeat Tom Corbett's assessment of carcinogenesis risk with better controls and anesthetic comparators. We didn't let on that we had nearly completed the study that we proposed. We had finished the exposures and sacrificed the mice. All that was left was completing the slides for histologic analysis and tabulating the results.

Jim Vitcha called me to request a small change in experimental design. TOO LATE! There was only one way to adequately explain why we couldn't accommodate his modest request: we had to confess our secret. Wendell and I flew to Chicago to meet with Jim, Ross, and other representatives of OMP. We took their scientists and executive team through our initial results. Our findings unambiguously exonerated isoflurane from any risk of carcinogenesis. We also exonerated four of the comparator anesthetics: enflurane, halothane, and nitrous oxide. The only anesthetic with a trace of suspicion, which did not reach statistical significance, was methoxyflurane.[21] Tom is a coauthor of this paper, reflecting my belief that science is well served when investigators collaborate.

After our presentation to OMP, Ross debriefed us on the internal corporate response. Evidently one of the lawyers complained to the management that Wendell and I had not done the study at the time and in the way OMP had requested. Ross remarked that such a complaint was like whining when you asked a batter to bunt and the batter hits a home run.

Isoflurane was approved in 1979. Enflurane and isoflurane added to the excellence of the drugs providing anesthesia. Like halothane, they did not explode. Clinically that's a big plus! They were unusually refractory to metabolism, nearly eliminating the risk of toxic metabolites. They offered other safety benefits over the previous generation of anesthetics, including better cardiovascular stability. They were less soluble than halothane, or methoxyflurane, resulting in more rapid onset and offset. This next generation of inhaled anesthetics provided clinicians with even greater precision in controlling the anesthetic state. Enflurane and isoflurane remained the primary inhaled anesthetics until the early 1990s.

The overwhelming dominance of isoflurane provided considerable revenue to OMP. In 1978, just before the approval of isoflurane, OMP was purchased by the British Oxygen Corporation (BOC Group). They moved the anesthetic products into a new division, Anaquest. The revenue from isoflurane radically decreased in the early 1990s when the patent expired. In 1993, Anaquest's assets were sold to Baxter.

The Continuing Search for a Better Anesthetic

Was there a better anesthetic to be discovered? A Japanese pharmaceutical company, Maruishi, thought they had the answer in sevoflurane (another compound synthesized by Ross) (**Figure 12.2**). Sevoflurane underwent significant

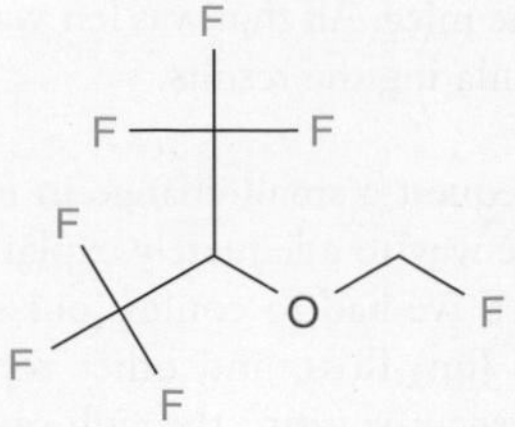

Figure 12.2   Sevoflurane.

metabolism, suggesting the possibility that sevoflurane would have clinical toxicity. Although there was no direct evidence for such toxicity, I wasn't very enthusiastic about seeing yet more metabolite toxicity, having seen how "halothane hepatitis" sidelined halothane a decade earlier. I wondered if there might be a better anesthetic among the other compounds in the 700 made and discarded by Ross.

Having helped identify the winning properties of isoflurane, I felt that I knew the profile of the next (and possibly best) anesthetic. Isoflurane set the bar so high that the next anesthetic would need to be nearly perfect. It would need to be halogenated only with fluorine, conferring metabolic stability. It would need to have no obvious adverse physiology. It would need to be even less soluble than isoflurane, conferring extremely rapid uptake and distribution, and precise control of anesthesia. Anaquest invited me to look at their inventory of molecules. We identified five candidates, but four were unstable in the presence of soda lime. We selected one, desflurane, for further study. Desflurane had the same structure as isoflurane, but with a chlorine replaced by fluorine (**Figure 12.3**).

Desflurane had a particular attraction for Anaquest. Desflurane was so difficult to synthesize that Anaquest had not bothered to patent it in the 1960s when it was made. They also hadn't published the structure, so there was no public disclosure. Thus, unlike sevoflurane, it could be developed with a full patent life.

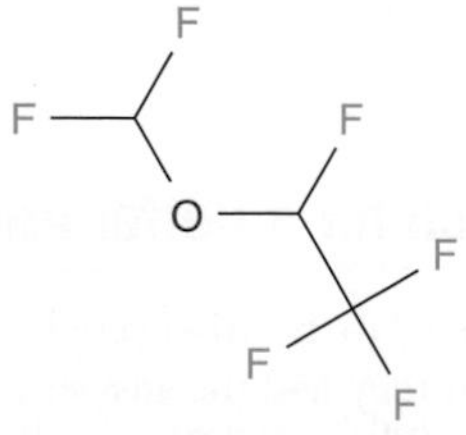

Figure 12.3   Desflurane.

Desflurane Versus Sevoflurane

By this time my laboratory at UCSF had been operating as an efficient machine for studying inhaled anesthetics for more than 2 decades. We trained our sights on desflurane, determined to dissect the clinical pharmacology in even greater detail than we had for its predecessors. Our studies of desflurane suggested that it had favorable properties. As anticipated, it had a low solubility,[22] a blood/gas partition coefficient of 0.45, and an associated rapid recovery from anesthesia in rats.[23] Low solubility in human tissues[24] and in the plastics and components of the anesthesia circuit anesthetic components[25] complimented the low blood/gas partition coefficient. Desflurane produced little or no toxicity when given with normal soda lime.[26,27] but was susceptible to degradation by dry soda lime.[28] Desflurane resisted metabolic degradation in rats.[29] Electroencephalographic changes in swine induced by anesthesia with desflurane paralleled those induced by isoflurane.[30] The cardiovascular effects of desflurane in swine were unremarkable.[31] Halogenation by fluorine produced a higher MAC in rats.[32] The only significant drawback for desflurane appeared to be the difficult synthesis. Our studies clearly showed that desflurane was a *new(!), better(!)* anesthetic, the inhaled anesthetic that the world was waiting for.

Although Ross had synthesized sevoflurane, Anaquest had sold the rights to sevoflurane. Eventually the rights were acquired by Maruishi for use in Japan, where they completed clinical development. Believing they had a winner, Maruishi offered to license the development and commercial use in the United States to Anaquest. However, Anaquest was certain from my research that desflurane was a far superior anesthetic. Anaquest did not have the resources to develop both anesthetics. Believing me, Anaquest refused the offer. Maruishi sold the rights to sevoflurane for use outside Japan to Abbott Pharmaceuticals. History would prove me wrong: sevoflurane was overwhelming adopted over desflurane as the best inhaled anesthetic (except at UCSF). I've accepted that conclusion.

As de facto medical director of Anaquest, but more importantly feeling a parental relationship to desflurane, I undertook studies that supplied the data needed to properly evaluate this new anesthetic and compare it to sevoflurane. Desflurane had the expected advantages vis-à-vis sevoflurane. Desflurane was less soluble, and thus had more rapid pharmacokinetics than sevoflurane. The kinetic advantages of desflurane provided a major reason for clinicians to prefer desflurane. Patients given desflurane woke up minutes sooner and under some conditions this provided a major reason for choosing desflurane. Desflurane also had superior chemical stability to sevoflurane. The liver left desflurane intact but degraded appreciable amounts of sevoflurane to potentially nephrotoxic fluorine. However, while this always remained a potential risk, clinical studies never showed evidence of kidney injury from sevoflurane. Soda lime degraded sevoflurane to compound A, a potent nephrotoxin. Here again sevoflurane was lucky; the production of compound A was never sufficient to cause clinically meaningful injury. My a priori concern about sevoflurane's lack of complete stability yielding toxic metabolites, or toxic degradation products, proved true. However, the actual clinical risk proved to be negligible.

There was one other risk with sevoflurane: explosion. The commonly used carbon dioxide absorbent Baralyme (but not soda lime) when desiccated could degrade sevoflurane to an explosive gaseous mixture. Abbott Laboratories, the purveyor of sevoflurane in the world outside of Japan, dealt effectively with this dramatic problem. After three cases of fire and/or explosion in circle absorption systems had been reported, Abbott eliminated the problem by buying the rights to Baralyme and taking it off the market.

However, desflurane had undesirable unforeseen traits, traits that could be controlled but required care to deal with smoothly. The primary problem was that at concentrations exceeding 1 MAC, desflurane could irritate the airway and stimulate the circulation. There was also an issue of drug delivery. Sevoflurane could be delivered in standard vaporizers. However, desflurane has a vapor pressure that approaches atmospheric pressure, and may boil at room temperature. To deliver a stable dose of anesthetic requires using a pressurized vaporizer. Additionally, desflurane is less potent than sevoflurane or isoflurane, and this requires more heat to vaporize an anesthetic concentration. By the time pressurized heated vaporizers for desflurane were available, sevoflurane had captured much of the market for the new, better anesthetic. Desflurane would always be more expensive because it was so hard to synthesize.

One other unforeseen advantage of sevoflurane might complete its sweep of the market. Sevoflurane and desflurane are both greenhouse gases. They block the escape of infrared light, contributing to global warming. However, desflurane may have an order of magnitude greater impact on infrared light and global warming than sevoflurane.[33,34] I hadn't thought to look at this when we evaluated desflurane in the early 1990s.

Something Better Than Desflurane and Sevoflurane?

My exploration of new inhaled anesthetics provides one more story. In 2007, I took another look at Ross' 700 compounds to see if I could find a competitor to desflurane and sevoflurane, an even better next anesthetic. As I noted earlier, there were several potential candidates, but most were unstable in the presence of soda lime. One of these was a sister to sevoflurane, identical to sevoflurane except for substitution of a fluorine for a hydrogen on the methyl moiety: $CHF_2-O-CH(CF_3)_2$. A less potent (MAC 8.3%) but much less soluble (blood/gas partition coefficient 0.21) sister to sevoflurane that unfortunately disintegrated in soda lime in tens of seconds. But what if we didn't use soda lime, an absorbent that contained a monovalent base? Would it still degrade so fast? I had a chemist friend make a batch of compound 15 (no, I don't remember why I called it that) and tested its stability in the absorbent Amsorb (no monovalent base). Perfectly stable! What excitement!

So, we anesthetized five volunteer rats with compound 15 and determined the MAC. As predicted, the rats recovered their righting reflexes more rapidly after anesthesia with compound 15 than after anesthesia with sevoflurane. But then we made one more test of rate of recovery, a more sensitive test, the rotarod test, a measure of the recovery of balance while walking. Rats anesthetized with compound 15 took significantly longer, much longer to recover than when anesthetized with sevoflurane. Damn! But why? We believe we know the answer although we didn't test our speculation. We believe compound 15 was much more vulnerable to metabolic degradation than sevoflurane. The product of degradation would be hexafluoroisopropanol $(HOC(CF_3)_2)$, a potent, lingering, highly soluble anesthetic.

Thus ended our search for a new, better, inhaled anesthetic. There may be one to be found, but I'm doubtful. I'm not sure that the world needs better anesthetics than sevoflurane and desflurane. These come very close to being perfect inhaled drugs. However, studying new inhaled anesthetics was so much fun that I didn't welcome turning off the lights on this party.

References

1. Saidman LJ, Eger EI II. Effect of nitrous oxide and of narcotic premedication on the alveolar concentration of halothane required for anesthesia. *Anesthesiology*. 1964;25:302-306.
2. Terrell RC, Speers L, Szur AJ, Treadwell J, Ucciardi TR. General anesthetics: 1. Halogenated methyl ethyl ethers as anesthetic agents. *J Med Chem*. 1971;14:517-519.
3. Stevens WC, Dolan WM, Gibbons RT, et al. Minimum alveolar concentrations (MAC) of isoflurane with and without nitrous oxide in patients of various ages. *Anesthesiology*. 1975;42:197-200.
4. Joas TA, Stevens WC, Eger EI II. Electroencephalographic seizure activity in dogs during anaesthesia. *Br J Anaesth*. 1971;43:739-745.
5. Cromwell TH, Stevens WC, Eger EI II, et al. The cardiovascular effects of compound 468 (Forane) during spontaneous ventilation and CO2 challenge in man. *Anesthesiology*. 1971;35:17-25.
6. Fourcade HE, Stevens WC, Larson CP Jr, et al. The ventilatory effects of Forane, a new inhaled anesthetic. *Anesthesiology*. 1971;35:26-31.

7. Hickey RF, Fourcade HE, Eger EI II, et al. The effects of ether, halothane, and Forane on apneic thresholds in man. *Anesthesiology.* 1971;35:32-37.

8. Eger EI II, Dolan WM, Stevens WC, Miller RD, Way WL. Surgical stimulation antagonizes the respiratory depression produced by Forane. *Anesthesiology.* 1972;36:544-549.

9. France CJ, Plumer HM, Eger EI II, Wahrenbrock EA. Ventilatory effects of isoflurane (Forane) or halothane when combined with morphine, nitrous oxide and surgery. *Br J Anaesth.* 1974;46:117-120.

10. Eger EI II, Stevens WC, Cromwell TH. The electroencephalogram in man anesthetized with Forane. *Anesthesiology.* 1971;35:504-508.

11. Miller RD, Eger EI II, Way WL, Stevens WC, Dolan WM. Comparative neuromuscular effects of Forane and halothane alone and in combination with d-tubocurarine in man. *Anesthesiology.* 1971;35:38-42.

12. Miller RD, Way WL, Dolan WM, Stevens WC, Eger EI II. The dependence of pancuronium- and d-tubocurarine-induced neuromuscular blockades on alveolar concentrations of halothane and Forane. *Anesthesiology.* 1972;37:573-581.

13. Vitez TS, Miller RD, Eger EI II, Van Nyhuis LS, Way WL. Comparison in vitro of isoflurane and halothane potentiation of d-tubocurarine and succinylcholine neuromuscular blockades. *Anesthesiology.* 1974;41:53-56.

14. Davison LA, Steinhelber JC, Eger EI II, Stevens WC. Psychological effects of halothane and isoflurane anesthesia. *Anesthesiology.* 1975;43:313-324.

15. Johnston RR, Eger EI II, Wilson C. A comparative interaction of epinephrine with enflurane, isoflurane, and halothane in man. *Anesth Analg.* 1976;55:709-712.

16. Halsey MJ, Sawyer DC, Eger EI II, Bahlman SH, Impelman DM. Hepatic metabolism of halothane, methoxyflurane, cyclopropane, Ethrane, and Forane in miniature swine. *Anesthesiology.* 1971;35:43-47.

17. Stevens WC, Eger EI, Joas TA, Cromwell TH, White A, Dolan WM. Comparative toxicity of isoflurane, halothane, fluroxene and diethyl ether in human volunteers. *Canad Anaesth Soc J.* 1973;20:357-368.

18. Dolan WM, Eger EI II, Margolis AJ. Forane increases bleeding in therapeutic suction abortion. *Anesthesiology.* 1972;36:96-97.

19. Johnson BH, Eger EI II. Bactericidal effects of anesthetics. *Anesth Analg.* 1979;58:136-138.

20. Corbett TH. Cancer and congenital anomalies associated with anesthetics. *Ann N Y Acad Sci.* 1976;271:58-66.

21. Eger EI, White AE, Brown CL, Biava CG, Corbett TH, Stevens WC. A test of the carcinogenicity of enflurane, isoflurane, halothane, methoxyflurane, and nitrous oxide in mice. *Anesth Analg.* 1978;57:678-694.

22. Eger EI II. Partition coefficients of I-653 in human blood, saline, and olive oil. *Anesth Analg.* 1987;66:971-973.

23. Eger EI II, Johnson BH. Rates of awakening from anesthesia with I-653, halothane, isoflurane, and sevoflurane: a test of the effect of anesthetic concentration and duration in rats. *Anesth Analg.* 1987;66:977-982.

24. Yasuda N, Targ AG, Eger EI II. Solubility of I-653, sevoflurane, isoflurane, and halothane in human tissues. *Anesth Analg.* 1989;69:370-373.

25. Targ AG, Yasuda N, Eger EI II. Solubility of I-653, sevoflurane, isoflurane, and halothane in plastics and rubber composing a conventional anesthetic circuit. *Anesth Analg.* 1989;69:218-225.

26. Eger EI II, Johnson BH, Ferrell LD. Comparison of the toxicity of I-653 and isoflurane in rats: a test of the effect of repeated anesthesia and use of dry soda lime. *Anesth Analg.* 1987;66:1230-1233.
27. Eger EI III. Stability of I-653 in soda lime. *Anesth Analg.* 1987;66:983-985.
28. Eger EI II, Strum DP. The absorption and degradation of isoflurane and I-653 by dry soda lime at various temperatures. *Anesth Analg.* 1987;66:1312-1315.
29. Koblin DD, Eger EI II, Johnson BH, Konopka K, Waskell L. I-653 resists degradation in rats. *Anesth Analg.* 1988;67:534-538.
30. Rampil IJ, Weiskopf RB, Brown JG, et al. I-653 and isoflurane produce similar dose-related changes in the electroencephalogram of pigs. *Anesthesiology.* 1988;69:298-302.
31. Weiskopf RB, Holmes MA, Eger EI II, Johnson BH, Rampil IJ, Brown JG. Cardiovascular effects of I-653 in swine. *Anesthesiology.* 1988;69:303-309.
32. Eger EI II, Johnson BH. MAC of I-653 in rats, including a test of the effect of body temperature and anesthetic duration. *Anesth Analg.* 1987;66:974-976.
33. Ryan SM, Nielsen CJ. Global warming potential of inhaled anesthetics: application to clinical use. *Anesth Analg.* 2010;111:92-98.
34. Sulbaek Andersen MP, Nielsen OJ, Wallington TJ, Karpichev B, Sander SP. Medical intelligence article: assessing the impact on global climate from general anesthetic gases. *Anesth Analg.* 2012;114:1081-1085.

Anesthetics and the Mind

13

Can Inhaled Anesthetics Permanently Change the Brain?

Anesthetics turn off the brain. At concentrations just slightly higher than anesthetic concentrations, the brain becomes isoelectric. *Ponder that for a moment—it's quite amazing! What other organ can we turn off and on in such a controlled manner?* Surely not the heart, the liver, or the kidney. *We can turn off, and then back on, not just any organ, but the human brain! Wow!*

Our ability to turn off brain electrical activity invites the question: is this OK? The profound central nervous system effects of anesthesia raise concern that some untoward residual effect remains after the drug has been eliminated by the body. This concern recurs in the history of anesthesia, despite the apparent absence of any expression of concern from Gilbert Abbott, the first publicly anesthetized patient. Despite lingering concerns, over the next 150 years only minor unpleasant effects (eg, nausea and vomiting) persisted once the anesthetic left the body. The possibility that subtle impairment of intelligence might occur and persist was largely ignored until recently when the possibility of risk to young children was raised.

However, I was troubled by the question. My laboratory at UCSF had developed sensitive assays for many of the physiologic effects of anesthetics, but our focus on the effects on the mind had been limited to simple responses to stimulation (eg, response to voice or something painful).

Such simple responses seemed inadequate to judge the effects of anesthesia on cognition. Developing such tests would allow us to look for subtle levels of cognitive impairment following recovery from anesthesia. In the early 1970s, we collaborated with two psychologists who were experts in cognitive assessment.[1] We gave 40 volunteers 1.0 to 2.0 MAC halothane or isoflurane for durations ranging from 4.4 to 8.6 hours, each with or without 70% nitrous oxide. We looked for evidence of cognitive or psychological changes before and 2, 4, 6, 8, and 30 days after anesthesia. We used long exposures to anesthesia because we knew that the effects would likely be subtle. Were there a clinically important effect, we would mostly likely see it with a long exposure.

We subjected 41 unanesthetized controls to the same measurements and compared results for differences between the control subjects and subjects anesthetized with various anesthetics. We found that changes in function were greatest 2 days after anesthesia. Cognitive function had returned to near preanesthesia values 8 days after anesthesia. Thirty days after anesthesia we found only slight symptom and mood effects, and no intellectual effect attributable to anesthesia. Halothane produced greater negative effects on moods and symptoms, and tended to produce greater negative effects on intellectual function, than did isoflurane.[1]

In sum, we found that prolonged and deeper levels of anesthesia can produce impaired cognition for up to 8 days after such anesthesia, and the choice of anesthetic may influence this effect. The study provided strong evidence that the effects of anesthesia on cognition were transient, and anesthetics did not produce lasting cognitive impairment.

What Inhaled Anesthetic Concentrations Change Brain Function?

The above studies in volunteers examined the effects of prolonged and profound anesthesia on psychological status and cognition, but they did not explore the effects of much smaller anesthetic concentrations. We knew nothing about trace exposure, the smallest concentration producing a measurable effect. Nor did they determine the residual concentration at which recovery is complete. I was worried about these, both because of the potential for harm to patients, but also because my colleagues and I spent every working day breathing trace concentrations of anesthetic drugs. Additionally, David Bruce and his colleagues had found evidence that trace concentrations[2,3] were associated with impaired cognition.

To examine the effects of trace anesthetics and collaborate or refute the findings of Bruce and colleagues, Tom Cook and I used three tests of mental function (choice-reaction time; digit span test; Purdue Pegboard Assembly test) in human volunteers breathing alveolar enflurane or halothane concentrations less than 0.1 MAC[4] or concentrations of halothane, nitrous oxide, or a combination of halothane and nitrous oxide less than 0.2 MAC.[5] These low concentrations had no effect on any of our sensitive measures of mental function. These results confirmed similar results published by Smith and Shirley shortly before we published our findings.[6] In my subsequent communications with David Bruce, he shared that his studies had experimental errors that he felt invalidated his results (D. Bruce, personal communication).

More than a decade later, about 1990, Hank Bennett called me. I didn't know Hank, we had never met, and I was not aware of his interests. However, Hank had heard me present our evidence that there were no residual long-term anesthetic effects on mentation. Hank didn't buy it. In his view, I had not used sufficiently sensitive measures of mental effects. Hank argued that I had ignored the possibility of long-term anesthetic effects on implicit (unconscious) memory. Sure, you can still drive a car, but can you still remember your violin lessons from third grade? Hank gradually convinced me that he might be correct. His arguments led to a productive collaboration that lasted a decade.

Rory Dwyer (**Figure 13.1**) led our first study, a study in which we measured MAC$_{awake}$. We provided our volunteers with answers to Trivial Pursuit-like questions (eg, what is the blood pressure of an octopus?).[7,8] When we gave the answers to such titillating questions to awake patients, those answers were nearly always remembered. However, when we gave answers to patients breathing 0.6 MAC or greater concentrations of isoflurane, nobody recalled them when asked later. They stopped responding to simple requests, such as "open your eyes." We also gave our modestly anesthetized patients suggestions for specific actions to undertake after they awoke. The anesthetized patients did not follow suggestions we gave them while anesthetized for things they should do when they awoke. Our team repeated the study with desflurane, with similar results.[9]

But there must be some subanesthetic concentration permitting the retention of information supplied. *What might that be?* We dared not study that in patients because it would not be acceptable to have patients awake during surgery. *However, we could study that in volunteers!*

And so we did. We found a 50% decrease in retention of Trivial Pursuit-like answers in subjects breathing 0.2 MAC isoflurane or 0.5 MAC nitrous oxide (**Figure 13.2**).[7] Thus, concentrations of isoflurane approaching trace anesthesia significantly suppressed memory, just as Hank had suspected. We also found that isoflurane caused more amnesia than nitrous oxide in terms of relative potency measured by MAC (**Figure 13.3**).

Remembering Relevant Versus Irrelevant Information

Hank still doubted the validity of our determination (**Figure 13.4**). *He was a tough guy to please!* Hank pointed to the problem presented by a study conducted by Levinson.[10] Levinson proposed that patients might not remember information supplied during anesthesia unless the information was relevant to their well-being. In other words, they might not retain the answers to stupid

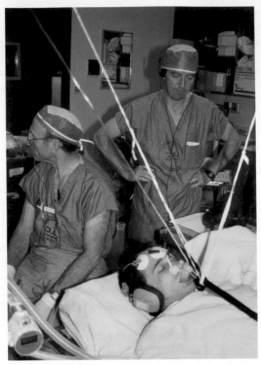

Figure 13.1   Me (seated), Rory Dwyer, and a volunteer receiving a subanesthetic concentration of nitrous oxide or isoflurane.

questions like the blood pressure of an octopus. However, it was possible that stating that a serious complication occurred that might result in death would leave an imprint in the patient's memory.

To test his thesis Levinson had studied 10 patients having ether anesthesia for dental procedures. The patients were anesthetized with ether, at a dose that caused EEG burst suppression (nearly flat EEG interrupted by bursts of electrical activity). Once anesthetized, each patient heard Levinson read a crisis script suggesting that the patient was at risk of not receiving sufficient oxygen, and that this required and received immediate correction. Thirty days after anesthesia, Levinson interviewed each patient and asked each if they remembered any events occurring during anesthesia. They did not, but under hypnosis, Levinson found that 4 of the 10 patients remembered verbatim portions of the crisis drama. Four other patients became apprehensive and broke out of the hypnotic trance.

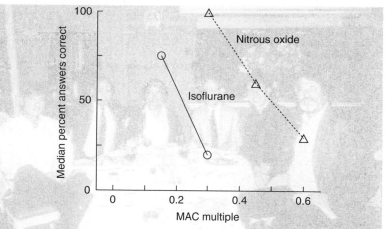

Figure 13.2 MAC multiples of nitrous oxide versus isoflurane to suppress recall of answers to trivial pursuit questions such as "where was Robert Redford born?" in volunteers. (From Dwyer R, Bennett HL, Eger El II, Heilbron D. Effects of isoflurane and nitrous oxide in subanesthetic concentrations on memory and responsiveness in volunteers. *Anesthesiology.* 1992;77:888-898.)

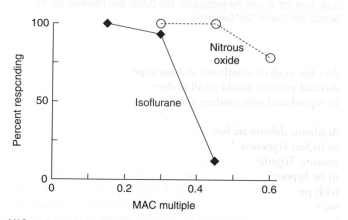

Figure 13.3 MAC$_{awake}$ in volunteers anesthetized with MAC multiples of nitrous oxide or isoflurane. (From Dwyer R, Bennett HL, Eger El II, Heilbron D. Effects of isoflurane and nitrous oxide in subanesthetic concentrations on memory and responsiveness in volunteers. *Anesthesiology.* 1992;77:888-898.)

This evidence supported Levinson's thesis. However, his experiment had several flaws and limitations. There was no control group. The study was not blinded. Levinson knew that each patient had received the crisis drama. Levinson supplied the hypnosis. Levinson interpreted the results. Finally, it was not clear that his study was even relevant, since ether is no longer used for anesthesia. Our

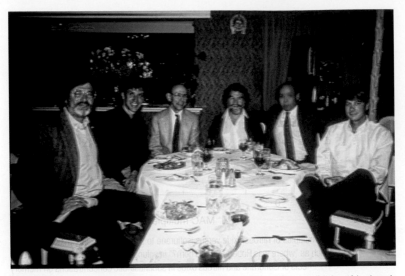

Figure 13.4   At the dinner celebrating the successful completion of the replication of Levinson's study, from left to right the participants: Bob Dutton, Ben Chortkoff, me, Bernard Levinson, Hank Bennett, and Charles "Ted" Gonsowski.

data for modern anesthetics did not support his findings that seemingly anesthetized patients would recall irrelevant information. Could Levinson's results be reproduced with modern anesthetics?

Academic debates are best settled by collaboration. We invited Levinson to join us in San Francisco. Levinson traveled from South Africa to participate in this venture. Together, we studied 21 volunteers, each selected for his or her capacity to be hypnotized. Each was anesthetized twice; once with desflurane and once with propofol. We first determined MAC$_{awake}$ in each subject. Following that, we tested each at 1.5 to 2 times his or her MAC$_{awake}$ value. The subject was randomized to hear a banal "drama" with one anesthetic and a crisis drama with the other anesthetic. The banal drama spoke to the excellence with which the study had proceeded. There was no emotional content. The crisis drama was terrifying—just writing it here makes me anxious:

> *"Oh, shit, who turned off the oxygen? Who disconnected the cylinder? Damn it, he's turned blue. God, his lips are blue. Get that thing connected again. You got it? O.K. I'm going to give him some more oxygen now. (15 seconds pause). Ho boy. O.K. He looks better now. I think we can continue."*

Both the banal and crisis dramas were presented through earphones that added concurrent room noises and conversations. The specific drama (banal or crisis) was not heard by the investigators in the room. Having been blinded to the drama, Levinson and Bennett interviewed the volunteer on the following day in an effort to determine which drama had been presented. A third blinded investigator, Block, viewed a video of the examination of each subject. During the interview, the investigators could ask the volunteer any question. They could hypnotize the volunteer to better determine which drama had been presented. After doing their best to gather information from the volunteer, they had to guess.

Their guesses were as correct as what one might expect by chance.[11] For example, Levinson guessed correctly in 11 of the 21 volunteers. Even with Levinson's help we could not replicate the results of his experiment. We do not know why we failed. Perhaps the presentation of our drama was less convincing—although one volunteer awoke after hearing the crisis drama and asked if something had gone wrong during his anesthesia. One strong possibility is that desflurane and propofol are much more potent amnestic drugs than is diethyl ether. However, blinding, the use of a control group, and the use of multiple investigators greatly reduced the possibility of our inserting unconscious bias into our experiment.

Awareness During Surgical Anesthesia

Several epidemiological studies have tested the incidence of awareness in patients given standard anesthetics (**Table 13.1**). The results are widely disparate. I believe three problems may have contributed to the disparities.

First, as we learned in our studies of awareness, there must be very tight control of the partial pressure administered to the patient. There is a dose-response relationship between anesthetic and consciousness. Our studies in volunteers show that too light a level increases the chance of awareness, just as one would expect. For example, recall is very high in trauma patients who receive reduced anesthetic doses.[17]

Second, the choice of anesthetic and the use of anesthetic adjuvants could affect the chance of awareness. Too great a reliance on nitrous oxide or opioids or neuromuscular blocking drugs will increase the likelihood of awareness. Conversely, potent amnestic drugs (benzodiazepines, propofol, and potent volatile anesthetics) will decrease awareness.

Third, and perhaps most likely, is that in these studies awareness appears based on subjective criteria that might not be widely accepted as suitable definitions. For example, one incidence of awareness was based on the patient's report of

Table 13.1 Reported Incidence of Awareness

Author	Year	Subjects	Age	Percent Aware
Sebel[12]	2004	19,575	Adult	0.13%
Ekman[13]	2004	7826	Adult	0.18%
Myles[14]	2004	1238	Adult	0.89%
Davidson[15]	2005	864	Child	0.81%
Pollard[16]	2007	87,361	Adult	0.0069%

an out-of-body experience.[12] Of note, the largest epidemiological study had the lowest incidence of awareness (6 out of 87,361 patients).[16] In Pollard's study, those who remembered a portion of their operation had received muscle relaxants. Of the six patients with awareness, four had undergone cardiac surgery, a procedure often associated with lighter levels of anesthesia.

But suppose that rare patients remember events under anesthesia despite maintenance of adequate surgical anesthesia with potent amnestic drugs given in what appear to be adequate amounts. *Why these patients and not others? What qualities are unique to these patients? Do they have a hidden history of exposure to depressant drugs (eg, alcohol) rendering them tolerant to anesthetics? Do they possess biochemical idiosyncrasies rendering them tolerant? Do unknown ventilation/perfusion abnormalities hide low blood concentrations of the anesthetic?* We don't know.

Why did I study awareness under anesthesia in the later portion of my professional career? Why do I spend several paragraphs in my autobiography describing the research of others in this topic?

I went into anesthesia for money and power. Remember? However, I was also motivated because I wanted to preclude the terror of being anesthetized, of losing control. That has been a fear of mine since childhood. When I needed a cholecystectomy in the early 1980s, I arranged to have it done under an epidural anesthetic. If an epidural was good enough for the Iowa farmer's wife, it was good enough for me, my decades of research into anesthetics notwithstanding. In the 2000s, I needed orthopedic procedures on a knee and a shoulder. Each operation was performed under regional anesthesia.

I am often critical of people who base important decisions on irrational fears. However, I'm one of them. Despite my decades of research demonstrating the safety of inhaled anesthetics, my fear of awareness under anesthesia has irrationally guided my personal medical decisions for anesthesia. Indeed, I think my fear has grown with age and the increasing threat of requiring surgery and anesthesia. Maybe I had more than a scientific interest in awareness during anesthesia.

Maybe I should be more understanding of irrational decisions by others.

References

1. Davison LA, Steinhelber JC, Eger EI II, Stevens WC. Psychological effects of halothane and isoflurane anesthesia. *Anesthesiology.* 1975;43:313-324.
2. Bruce DL, Bach MJ, Arbit J. Trace anesthetic effects on perceptual, cognitive, and motor skills. *Anesthesiology.* 1974;40:453-458.
3. Bruce DL, Bach MJ. Psychological studies of human performance as affected by traces of enflurane and nitrous oxide. *Anesthesiology.* 1975;42:194-205.
4. Cook TL, Smith M, Winter PM, Starkweather JA, Eger EI II. Effect of subanesthetic concentrations of enflurane and halothane on human behavior. *Anesth Analg.* 1978;57:434-440.
5. Cook TL, Smith M, Starkweather JA, Winter PM, Eger EI II. Behavioral effects of trace and subanesthetic halothane and nitrous oxide in man. *Anesthesiology.* 1978;49:419-424.
6. Smith G, Shirley AW. Failure to demonstrate effect of trace concentrations of nitrous oxide and halothane on psychomotor performance. *Br J Anaesth.* 1977;49:65-70.
7. Dwyer R, Bennett HL, Eger EI II, Heilbron D. Effects of isoflurane and nitrous oxide in subanesthetic concentrations on memory and responsiveness in volunteers. *Anesthesiology.* 1992;77:888-898.
8. Dwyer R, Bennett HL, Eger EI II, Peterson N. Isoflurane anesthesia prevents unconscious learning. *Anesth Analg.* 1992;75:107-112.
9. Gonsowski CT, Chortkoff BS, Eger EI II, Bennett HL, Weiskopf RB. Subanesthetic concentrations of desflurane and isoflurane suppress explicit and implicit learning. *Anesth Analg.* 1995;80:568-572.
10. Levinson BW. States of awareness during general anaesthesia. Preliminary communication. *Br J Anaesth.* 1965;37:544-546.
11. Chortkoff BS, Gonsowski CT, Bennett HL, et al. Subanesthetic concentrations of desflurane and propofol suppress recall of emotionally charged information. *Anesth Analg.* 1995;81:728-736.
12. Sebel PS, Bowdle TA, Ghoneim MM, et al. The incidence of awareness during anesthesia: a multicenter United States study. *Anesth Analg.* 2004;99:833-839.
13. Ekman A, Lindholm ML, Lennmarken C, Sandin R. Reduction in the incidence of awareness using BIS monitoring. *Acta Anaesthesiol Scand.* 2004;48:20-26.
14. Myles PS, Leslie K, McNeil J, Forbes A, Chan MT. Bispectral index monitoring to prevent awareness during anaesthesia: the B-Aware randomised controlled trial. *Lancet.* 2004;363:1757-1763.
15. Davidson AJ, Huang GH, Czarnecki C, et al. Awareness during anesthesia in children: a prospective cohort study. *Anesth Analg* 2005;100:653-661, table of contents.
16. Pollard RJ, Coyle JP, Gilbert RL, Beck JE. Intraoperative awareness in a regional medical system: a review of 3 years' data. *Anesthesiology.* 2007;106:269-274.
17. Bogetz MS, Katz JA. Recall of surgery for major trauma. *Anesthesiology.* 1984;61:6-9.

MAC and Theories of Narcosis

14

MAC Soon Connected to Theories of Narcosis

How do inhaled anesthetics work? We understand the answer at a pharmacokinetic level. Anesthetics diffuse from the lungs into the blood, and from the blood into neuronal tissue. We understand the answer at a pharmacodynamic level. Anesthetics suppress the body's response to noxious stimulation. They suppress the brain's ability to form memories. They suppress consciousness, rendering patients oblivious to surgery. We understand the processes of uptake and distribution. We understand the clinical responses to anesthetic drugs. We can answer the "how" question with sufficient precision to safely use the drugs to induce the remarkable state of general anesthesia.

Despite the vast amount that we do understand, we simply don't know how inhaled anesthetics work. The above practical explanation of "how they work" doesn't explain how anesthetics interact with neural tissue to render the patient still ("immobile") when the surgeon cuts through the flesh. Where, exactly, does that happen? How, exactly, does that happen? By what pharmacological mechanism do inhaled anesthetics induce seemingly magical lack of responsiveness?

As discussed in Chapters 6 and 7, Giles Merkel and I described MAC as the potency of inhaled anesthetic that prevents response to painful stimulus in dogs.[1] Later, Larry Saidman and I described the same concept in humans.[2] Remarkably, the value of MAC was the same for dogs and humans. Given that we are so much smarter than dogs, why do our brains blink off at the same concentration that renders a dog immobile in response to noxious stimulation? It turns out that it's not just humans and dogs that can be anesthetized. Nearly all living organisms can be "anesthetized" within a surprisingly narrow concentration range.[3,4]

To understand how anesthetics work, we looked for factors that affected MAC. Of course, this information was clinically important to safe anesthesia. However, identifying factors that affected MAC might also give us insight into how anesthetics work. We found that MAC was an absolute partial pressure, not a fraction of inspired air.[5] That showed that inhaled anesthetics were acting as drugs with dose versus response relationships that had nothing to do with the air that the patient was breathing.

One of our most intriguing findings from that time was the correlation of MAC with the lipophilicity of the anesthetic, ie, the ability of anesthetic gas to dissolve in oil.[6] The question goes back to the observation Meyer[7] and Overton[8] described in Chapter 7 that lipophilicity (the ability of an anesthetic to dissolve in oil) was correlated with anesthetic potency **over five orders of magnitude** (see Figure 7.3). What does this mean? The correlation is too good, the span is too large, to be mere coincidence. John Severinghaus again provided the nidus: did lipophilicity correlate with our measurements of potency using MAC? It did (see Figure 7.2).[6] Could this tell us something about how anesthetics work?

We found that the MAC of halothane and cyclopropane correlated directly with changes in body temperature.[9] We noted that "*The heat changes (enthalpies) calculated from these data correlated well with enthalpies of absorption of anesthetics to lipoprotein films. In the case of cyclopropane they also correlated well with the enthalpies found for hydrate formation from ice.*" Pauling[10] and Miller[11] had recently proposed that anesthesia resulted from the formation of hydrates or ice crystals at neuronal surfaces. Our calculations supported their theory, now long discarded and only of historical interest.

Using MAC as our measure of anesthetic potency, we probed for deviations from the correlation of lipophilicity and potency. We only found a few slight exceptions.[12] As Koblin noted, "The product of the anesthetizing partial pressure of an agent and its oil-gas partition coefficient varies less than twofold over a 70,000-fold range of anesthetic partial pressures."[13] The exceedingly lipophilic anesthetic thiomethoxyflurane (oil/gas partition coefficient 7230) had a correspondingly small MAC of 0.035% atm.[14] Like the Meyer-Overton "theory," the correlation of MAC with lipophilicity withstood extreme tests of the correlation.

The precise correlation of lipophilicity and potency, and the constancy of the product of lipophilicity × potency, supported the notion that inhaled anesthetics acted by their presence in lipid. Perhaps this was the lipid deep within the membrane bilayer. It might be lipid within some hydrophobic (water-repelling) portion of a neuronal protein. We were convinced that knowing where to look, the lipophilic regions of neurons, would readily take us to the answer. Most likely there was a simple answer that would, in retrospect, be obvious. All we needed was that "ah ha!" moment when someone would say "couldn't this all be explained by X?" We would test X, and this hundred-year-old puzzle would be solved.

We and others had our "ah ha" moments. Many of them. None led to the answer. We dug deeper and deeper, ruling out theory after theory.[15] The more we learned, the greater the mystery.

Exceptions to the Correlation of MAC and Lipophilicity

In the early 1990s, we further tested the correlation of MAC and lipophilicity by examining properties of progressively larger n-alkanes. These are straight chain organic molecules, such as methane (one carbon), ethane (two carbons), propane (three carbons), and n-butane (four carbons). These are all anesthetics. We hoped that by merely expanding chain length we could garner insights into where they were acting.

As expected from basic organic chemistry, lipophilicity progressively increased with increasing carbon chain length. However, to our surprise, the tight correlation between anesthetic potency and lipophilicity fell apart when the carbon chain exceeded six.[16] Above this chain length, the product of potency and lipophilicity was no longer constant, but progressively increased. Increase in chain length also correlated with a decrease in hydrophilicity (ie, a decreased saline/gas partition coefficient). The largest alkane we tested was n-decane, a chain of 10 carbons.

In the succeeding year, we tested perfluorinated (completely fluorinated) alkanes. These are more clinically relevant because they don't blow up the way that, say, butane might. As expected, the simplest perfluorinated alkane, CF_4, had anesthetic effects. Unexpectedly, neither C_2F_6, just one carbon longer, nor longer elements of the series had any anesthetic effects despite lipophilicity suggesting anesthetic potency.[17] If the lack of anesthetic effect was simply caused by replacing hydrogen with fluorine, then we could try some "in between" molecules that were only partly fluorinated. Wrong again! A subsequent study of partially fluorinated alkanes, alkanes having up to six carbons, revealed that partly replacing hydrogen with fluorine could not explain the breakdown in correlation between lipophilicity and potency.[18]

It appeared that the Meyer-Overton correlation was flawed. *Perhaps we had been looking in the wrong place!* Perhaps a hydrophobic (lipophilic) site was not necessarily where anesthetics acted.

One unexpected result from my collaboration with Ohio Medical Products was the finding of poor anesthetics. It isn't surprising that in our search for better anesthetics we stumbled across a couple of losers. In this case, the losers did not produce anesthesia despite having a lipophilicity that predicted that they should be good anesthetics. A few decades later, we realized that these "losers" might be powerful research tools. An absence of anesthetic effect might be a powerful tool for investigating how anesthetics work.

We had identified five alkanes with various hydrogen-halogen substitutions that had no capacity to produce immobility in the face of noxious stimulation despite what would appear to be adequate lipophilicity.[19] We initially called these five compounds nonanesthetics but changed that to nonimmobilizers when it was discovered that they might have the capacity to impair memory, to cause amnesia.[20] We also identified nine polyhalogenated alkanes that were much less potent than their lipophilicity predicted. We called these transitional compounds because their anesthetic potency lay between those of an immobilizer (conventional anesthetic) and those of a nonimmobilizer (zero potency). What distinguished the nonimmobilizers and, to a lesser extent, distinguished the transitional compounds was their diminished affinity to water, a low saline/gas partition coefficient. Compounds without anesthetic effect had remarkably small saline/gas partition coefficients. To further examine the importance of aqueous affinity to potency, we measured the MAC of n-alkanols: methanol, ethanol, butanol, hexanol, and octanol. Alkanols have far greater saline/gas partition coefficients than clinically used inhaled anesthetics. We found that MAC was roughly an order of magnitude greater than their lipophilicity would predict.[21] Here was an "*ah ha!*" moment: molecules with significant deviations from Meyer-Overton. Surely these would lead us to the answer!

Anesthesia Requires Both Lipophilicity and Hydrophilicity

Our studies of lipophilicity and hydrophilicity showed that anesthetics required both properties. In other words, they had to be amphipathic. This substantially narrowed our search for the site of anesthetic action: the site had to have both lipid and aqueous characteristics. This effectively ruled out the possibility that anesthetics act within the membrane bilayer because there is no water in the bilayer. However, they could act at the membrane's surface, the interface between membrane and extracellular or intracellular water. At these locations, anesthetics could have one foot in lipid and the other in water. In fact, simulations of anesthetic properties in the water-fat interface of bilayers predicted the observed cutoff.[22]

This was getting confusing! I reached out to experts from a number of fields, offering them fame and research funding if they could help me find the lipid-aqueous site where anesthetics acted. We created a Program Project and applied to the National Institutes of Health for multimillion-dollar support for our study "Sites and Mechanisms of Anesthetic Actions." I became the Director of this Program Project that continued from 1994 to 2009. It was a 15-year endeavor that linked some of the cleverest people in the field, who brought the best science available to my passionate pursuit of the mechanism of inhaled anesthesia. Our earliest studies supported our conclusion that anesthetics must be amphipathic (ie, parts of the molecule want to be in water, and other parts want to be in fat).[23,24]

We used our transitional compounds and nonimmobilizers to test various theories of narcosis. Frank and Loeb had suggested a decade earlier that anesthetics should have receptors on proteins, just like nearly every other drug.[25] That appeared to be a good place to start, so we used our transitional compounds and nonimmobilizers to look at specific receptors.

$GABA_A$ and glycine receptors are putative mediators. Both are inhibitory in action. An anesthetic would be expected to (and does) enhance the responses of these receptors to their endogenous ligands, GABA and glycine. Do they respond as predicted to anesthetics versus nonimmobilizers? Transitional and nonimmobilizer compounds should have less or no effect on these receptors. That is what we found for $GABA_A$ receptors.[26] However, in subsequent experiments, we proved that neither $GABA_A$ nor glycine receptors could be mediators of immobility.[27]

I found our investigation of fluorinated alkanes that had a single hydrogen at either end to be exciting in its implications. An increase in chain length up to four carbons progressively increased anesthetic potency, but compounds six or more carbons in length were nonimmobilizers. I suggested that one interpretation of this finding was that anesthetics produce immobility by acting on two sites approximately five carbons apart.[28] Subsequent structure-activity relationship (SAR) modeling suggested that this observation is consistent with the known structures of volatile anesthetics and predicts nonimmobilizers.[29]

Our 15 years of NIH-funded research was highly productive. Greg Homanics, one of our coinvestigators, created murine strains with mutations in the $GABA_A$, NMDA, and glycine receptors to help dissect their contributions to anesthetic action. We also had access to mice strains with mutated sodium channels. Other coinvestigators (Jim Sonner, Mike Fanselow, Adron Harris, Bob Pearce, and Misha Perouansky) studied how these knock-in and knock-out mutations altered anesthetic pharmacology. Meanwhile, Joe Antognini and his colleagues tried to find the spinal circuitry responsibility for immobility. We produced nearly 100 papers in the final grant period alone (2005-2009), ruling out nearly all of the possible synaptic targets.[15]

Despite the intellectual firepower assembled for our Program Project, despite having access to the best available tools of neuroscience and molecular biology, we never found the answer. This still unanswered question inspired my research until my ninth decade. I have few regrets, but one is that I will never know how inhaled anesthetics accomplish their magic.

The "*ah ha!*" moment, the thrill of solving the hardest puzzle in all of pharmacology, awaits another investigator.

References

1. Merkel G, Eger EI II. A comparative study of halothane and halopropane anesthesia including method for determining equipotency. *Anesthesiology*. 1963;24:346-357.

2. Saidman LJ, Eger EI II. Effect of nitrous oxide and of narcotic premedication on the alveolar concentration of halothane required for anesthesia. *Anesthesiology*. 1964;25:302-306.

3. Sonner JM. A hypothesis on the origin and evolution of the response to inhaled anesthetics. *Anesth Analg*. 2008;107:849-854.

4. Eckenhoff RG. Why can all of biology be anesthetized? *Anesth Analg*. 2008;107:859-861.

5. Eger EI II, Saidman LJ, Brandstater B. Minimum alveolar anesthetic concentration: a standard of anesthetic potency. *Anesthesiology*. 1965;26:756-763.

6. Eger EI II, Brandstater B, Saidman LJ, Regan MJ, Severinghaus JW, Munson ES. Equipotent alveolar concentrations of methoxyflurane, halothane, diethyl ether, fluroxene, cyclopropane, xenon and nitrous oxide in the dog. *Anesthesiology*. 1965;26:771-777.

7. Meyer HH. Theorie der Alkoholnarkose. *Arch Exptl Pathol Pharmakol*. 1899;42:109-118.

8. Overton E. *Studien über die Narkose, Zugleich ein Beitrag zur allgemeinen Pharmakologie*. Gustav Fischer; 1901:1-195.

9. Eger EI II, Saidman LJ, Brandstater B. Temperature dependence of halothane and cyclopropane anesthesia in dogs: correlation with some theories of anesthetic action. *Anesthesiology*. 1965;26:764-770.

10. Pauling L. A molecular theory of anesthesia. *Science*. 1961;134:15-21.

11. Miller SL. Theory of gaseous anesthetics. *Proc Natl Acad Sci USA*. 1961;47:1515-1524.

12. Targ AG, Yasuda N, Eger EI II, et al. Halogenation and anesthetic potency. *Anesth Analg*. 1989;68:599-602.

13. Koblin DD, Eger EI. Current concepts: theories of narcosis. *N Engl J Med*. 1979;301:1222-1224.

14. Tanifuji Y, Eger EI II, Terrell RC. Some characteristics of an exceptionally potent inhaled anesthetic: thiomethoxyflurane. *Anesth Analg*. 1977;56:387-390.

15. Eger EI II, Raines DE, Shafer SL, Hemmings HC Jr, Sonner JM. Is a new paradigm needed to explain how inhaled anesthetics produce immobility? *Anesth Analg*. 2008;107:832-848.

16. Taheri S, Laster MJ, Liu J, Eger EI II, Halsey MJ, Koblin DD. Anesthesia by n-alkanes not consistent with the Meyer-Overton hypothesis: determinations of the solubilities of alkanes in saline and various lipids. *Anesth Analg.* 1993;77:7-11.

17. Liu J, Laster MJ, Koblin DD, et al. A cut-off in potency exists in the perfluoroalkanes. *Anesth Analg.* 1994;79:238-244.

18. Eger EI II, Liu J, Koblin DD, et al. Molecular properties of the "ideal" inhaled anesthetic: studies of fluorinated methanes, ethanes, propanes, and butanes. *Anesth Analg.* 1994;79:245-251.

19. Koblin DD, Chortkoff BS, Laster MJ, Eger EI II, Halsey MJ, Ionescu P. Polyhalogenated and perfluorinated compounds that disobey the Meyer-Overton hypothesis. *Anesth Analg.* 1994;79:1043-1048.

20. Kandel L, Chortkoff BS, Sonner J, Laster MJ, Eger EI II. Nonanesthetics can suppress learning. *Anesth Analg.* 1996;82:321-326.

21. Fang ZX, Ionescu P, Chortkoff BS, et al. Anesthetic potencies of n-alkanols: results of additivity studies suggest a mechanism of action similar to that for conventional inhaled anesthetics. *Anesth Analg.* 1997;84:1042-1048.

22. Cantor RS. Breaking the Meyer-Overton rule: predicted effects of varying stiffness and interfacial activity on the intrinsic potency of anesthetics. *Biophys J.* 2001;80:2284-2297.

23. Pohorille A, Wilson MA. Excess chemical potential of small solutes across water-membrane and water-hexane interfaces. *J Chem Phys.* 1996;104:3760-3773.

24. Chipot C, Wilson MA, Pohorille A. Interactions of anesthetics with the water-hexane interface. A molecular dynamics study. *J Phys Chem B.* 1997;101:782-791.

25. Franks NP, Lieb WR. Do general anaesthetics act by competitive binding to specific receptors? *Nature.* 1984;310:599-601.

26. Mihic SJ, McQuilkin SJ, Eger EI II, Ionescu P, Harris RA. Potentiation of gamma-aminobutyric acid type A receptor-mediated chloride currents by novel halogenated compounds correlates with their abilities to induce general anesthesia. *Mol Pharmacol.* 1994;46:851-857.

27. Zhang Y, Wu S, Eger EI II, Sonner JM. Neither GABA(A) nor strychnine-sensitive glycine receptors are the sole mediators of MAC for isoflurane. *Anesth Analg.* 2001;92:123-127.

28. Eger EI II, Halsey MJ, Harris RA, et al. Hypothesis: volatile anesthetics produce immobility by acting on two sites approximately five carbons apart. *Anesth Analg.* 1999;88:1395-1400.

29. Sewell JC, Sear JW. Determinants of volatile general anesthetic potency: a preliminary three-dimensional pharmacophore for halogenated anesthetics. *Anesth Analg.* 2006;102:764-771.

Epilogue 15

Epiphanies

My life changed course several times, evolving consequent to life circumstances. I found epiphanies in unexpected places. The discovery of reading at the age of 3 years blew my little mind, changing my world forever. Selling shoes one evening at Maling's was an epiphany. It convinced me that I wanted no part of selling shoes as my life's work, and that I might do just that if I continued to fail as a student. I completely reversed my academic trajectory after that evening, substituting persistence for intellectual firepower. My academic standing improved, and enabled my admittance to medical school.

Having entered medical school, I intended to become a general practitioner who in his spare time would make discoveries parallel to those made by Pasteur or Koch. Yeah, right…

I was young. I didn't realize that the days of Pasteur and Koch were gone. There was no chance I could have succeeded in emulating such men in their great discoveries. Fortunately, I was rescued from a lifetime of disappointment by another epiphany. In the summer after completing my first year of medical school, I discovered how easily an anesthetist might kill a patient. If I made anesthesia my career, every day I could take a patient's life in my hands. The possibility was overwhelmingly attractive.

So, into anesthesia I went. During my 1956 to 1958 residency another life-changing event arrived unexpectedly. I attended a lecture by John Severinghaus on the movement of anesthetics into the body. Fascinating! Compelling! Challenging! And (best of all) doable! John didn't appreciate all the nuances in pharmacokinetics. Arrogantly, I thought I could figure it out and tell the world of my brilliant insights with just a few months of study. Decades later I was still dotting "i"s and crossing "t"s.

My fascination with anesthetic uptake and distribution led to a fellowship in 1960 with John at the University of California at San Francisco (UCSF). That fellowship led to John's fateful request that I evaluate a new inhaled anesthetic, halopropane. To do that I had to discover MAC, a fundamental property of all inhaled anesthetics.

I was afforded an opportunity to experimentally validate my concepts of uptake and distribution and expand them with new research tools. That opened the door to a lifetime quantifying the effects and consequences of anesthesia.

My lovely wife, Lynn, thinks these are discoveries parallel to those of Pasteur and Koch. She thinks I've accomplished my naïve dreams of glory. She is wildly and dearly biased, but I still love hearing her attest to my brilliance.

Family

My first marriage to Dollie ended in divorce, and, in the good Jewish tradition, I felt guilty for the pain it caused her. But the marriage resulted in four wonderful children whom I love dearly. After 15 years alone (sort of—with various women), I met and married Lynn Spitler, who contributed two more children to our fold. As described in Chapter 11, our families combined well together, sharing love, generosity, and kindness for one another. As I approach my 10th decade, I am glad my wife, Lynn, is at my side.

Connections With the World

The fellowship with John completely changed my life. In bringing me to UCSF, John opened the door to one of the greatest medical research institutions. The Department of Anesthesia had access to world-class resources, faculty, and fellows. Membership in the UCSF faculty led to support as a fellow under the Department of Anesthesia's training grant and to a Research Career Development Award in the 1960s. Additionally, Bill Hamilton, Chair of the Department, directed a Program Project Grant that generously funded my research in the 1960s and 1970s. That support led to 25 years of Program Project Grants that I directed—10 years devoted to Aging and Anesthesia, and 15 years to Mechanisms of Inhaled Anesthetic Actions, including how these anesthetics impaired memory.

The UCSF connection and my fame as a leading investigator led to financial support by Ohio Medical Products and its successors. Ohio Medical Products also gave me access to compounds and collaborations with their scientists. My collaboration with Ross Terrell led to our establishing the standards by which modern inhaled anesthetics were developed, clinically evaluated, and used in the practice of anesthesia.

My research with numerous collaborators has led to over 500 peer-reviewed publications, including 9 of 100 Citation Classics, and numerous awards, including the ASA Distinguished Service Award and the ASA Excellence in Research Award. The coauthors on these publications included fellows who subsequently became two medical school deans, four ASA Distinguished Service Awardees, four ASA Excellence in Research Awardees, and 24 Department Chairs (US). They included Editors-in-Chief of Anesthesiology and of Anesthesia and Analgesia and nine American Board of Anesthesiology Directors. Following their fellowships, my fellows published over 1600 of their own papers.

I continue to participate in lectures to the incoming Anesthesia Residents on the topics of uptake and distribution and the history of anesthesia. I enjoy this interaction, and they have uniformly given me high marks for these talks. The Class of 2018 insisted on having their picture taken with me (**Figure 15.1**) and presented me with a framed copy of the picture and a cup with the picture on it (which I requested when they asked me what I would like as a tribute).

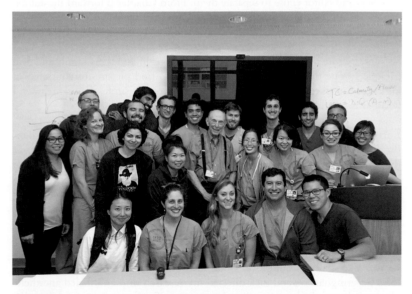

Figure 15.1   Photo of me with the UCSF Anesthesia Class of 2018 following my lecture on uptake and distribution of anesthetics. Front row: (from left) Jane Yu, Marci Pepper, Alison Schultz, Michael Lubrano, and Michael Wu. Second row: Tina Yu, Angela Wight, Revati Nafday, Esther Lee, me, Anne Park, Lisa Sun, and Ana Valdez. Third row: Scott Grubb, Alec Peniche, Jason Lang, Robert Caughey, Vikram Fielding-Singh, Andrew Bishara, C. Phillip Aguilar, and Thanh-Giang (Tina) Vu. Back row: Sandeep Sabhlok, and K. Elliot Higgins.

I Wrote This for You

Why would anyone want to read my autobiography? When Lynn, my children, and my close friends encouraged my writing this, I asked who might want to read it. The not-too-reassuring response was "we would." Well, OK. To my wife, my children, and my close friends: Here it is. I wrote this for you.

However, my guess is that my wife, family, and close friends will be perplexed why I devote so much of the text to the science of anesthetic pharmacology. Why delve into MAC, pharmacokinetics, and mechanisms of anesthetic action in such detail? There are two reasons.

First, this is my story. This science, in all its gritty detail, is inseparable from my life. There is a phrase, "*love me, love my dog.*" My version would be "*love me, love my science.*" The science of my life is so interwoven with my personal and family life that my original text mixed my scientific and personal stories in every chapter. My reviewers and editor chose to separate them. From Chapter 6 forward the autobiography bifurcates the scientific and personal stories into separate chapters. Maybe it is easier to read that way, but it isn't how I wrote it. To me they are all one story.

Second, I wrote this for you. My hope is that "you" includes my family and dear friends. I hope that leafing through the pages to find pictures of yourselves as kids is as fun to read as it was to write. If it makes you smile, then remember, I wrote this for you.

I also hope that "you" includes the next generation of anesthesia researchers. By sharing my story, I want to offer an example of the struggles, and rewards, that await you. I have already spoken of the lesson I learned as an inferior student struggling to improve my academic record. *Persistence!* Again, quoting Coolidge, "*Persistence and determination alone are omnipotent.*" That's close, but it is not the full story. More than persistence is required.

Luck is required. Good luck brought me to Lloyd Gittleson and Gwen Gleave at Grant Hospital in Chicago, where I learned from two masters that anesthesia was a specialty I could love. Good luck brought me to Iowa, where I met John Severinghaus. Good luck directed my research into an inhaled anesthetic pharmacology, which was undergoing a wave of commercial innovation that provided relevance and funding for my studies into the concepts of MAC and anesthetic pharmacokinetics. I am grateful for my good fortune. But for luck, things would have turned out very differently, and probably for the worse.

Mentorship is required. John Severinghaus brought incredible mentorship, both intellectually and culturally. His keen mind posed challenging questions, sparking many of my studies. However, culturally he was happy to play a supporting role, rather than demanding that my work serve to advance his career. John let me quickly break free and run with the ideas and experiments to build my own career. Every mentor can learn from John's example.

A supportive environment is required. I had the good fortune that my career led me to the Department of Anesthesia at UCSF. At that time, UCSF was emerging as one of the premier academic anesthesia departments in the world. I had laboratory space, protected time for research, and access to some of the finest minds in research. Persistence cannot overcome an inhospitable research environment.

If you are a young anesthesiologist contemplating a career in investigation, then the lesson I hope you take from this book is that you need a lifetime of persistence, a great mentor, a great environment, and some good luck. *If these come together for you, then I hope you can tell the world, and perhaps me, how general anesthetics work their magic!* Please do because I wrote this for you.

If you are a young anesthesiologist who is not interested in research, then I hope the chapters on MAC and pharmacokinetics will deepen your understanding of the clinical concepts that govern inhaled anesthetic pharmacology. The frontiers of science have long since moved on. However, these concepts remain one of the foundations of clinical practice. Perhaps the dense, detailed chapters on MAC and pharmacokinetics, placed in the context of my passion for anesthesia, will make them easier to understand and incorporate into your practice. If so, I wrote this for you.

Ida Beam, the Ether Dome, and The Wondrous Story of Anesthesia

In 1995, John Tinker, an old friend and Chairman of the Department of Anesthesia at the University of Iowa, invited me to give a lecture on the history of anesthesia. Not just any lecture, the university-wide Ida Beam Lecture. This lecture honored Ida Beam, a farmer's wife who literally gave the farm to the University of Iowa, a school she had not attended, but clearly admired. The University sold the farm and created an endowed lectureship in her honor.

"John, why me, and why the history of anesthesia, a subject to which I may have contributed but about which I know little?" *"Easy"* said John. *"1996 is the dual sesquicentennial of the discovery of anesthesia and the founding of the University. And the Dean has asked for this talk in which you would interconnect the two events. You're one of our bright graduates and you talk good."* Who could resist? Not many have been the Ida Beam lecturer.

Somehow I found the story of the history of anesthesia in Thorwald's book, *The Century of the Surgeon*.[1] A fifth of the book gives a fictional narrative of the history of anesthesia as seen through the eyes of a surgical resident. It took some liberties with the story and I gradually discovered those fictions, but it told an exciting tale that I used for my sesquicentennial talk.

I read more, learned more, corrected most of my misapprehensions. I gave the talk again and again, a talk that with time came closer to the truth. I was asked to speak at Harvard and accepted with the understanding that I would speak on the history of anesthesia and would do so in the Ether Dome.

In 1997 I did just that (**Figure 15.2**). With my daughter (Renee), Lynn, and author Julie Fenster (who had written a book focused on Morton's demonstration),[2] I stood where Morton had stood more than 150 years earlier in his great moment (**Figure 15.3**).

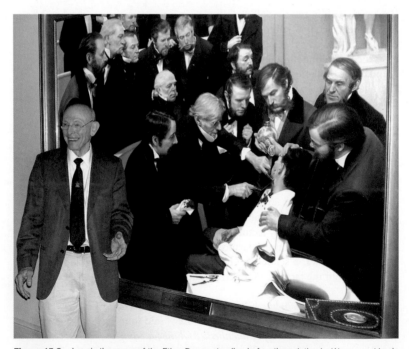

Figure 15.2   I am in the arena of the Ether Dome, standing before the painting by Warren and Lucia Prosperi depicting the first public demonstration of anesthesia, John Collin Warren's resection of Gilbert Abbott's lesion.

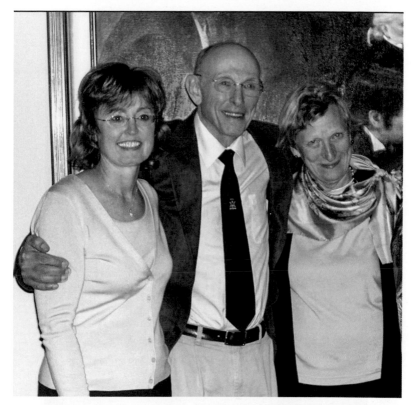

Figure 15.3 My daughter Renee, me, and my wife, Lynn, standing before Warren and Lucia Prosperi's depiction in the Ether Dome of the first successful demonstration of anesthesia.

Books I Have Authored

I have authored seven books and authored or coauthored 53 book chapters. Three of the authored books were/are of particular importance. The first of these, *Anesthetic Uptake and Action*,[3] resulted from more than a decade of study and described what was known about inhaled anesthetic pharmacokinetics in the early 1970s (**Figure 15.4**). Although it is nearly a half century old and has no information on the most modern potent inhaled anesthetics, the principles it describes are relevant today. I have wanted to produce an updated edition for decades. I recently completed my chapters for the second edition, adding sevoflurane and desflurane. It remains to be seen whether my unnamed coauthor will complete his chapters, allowing the second edition to be published. No pressure!

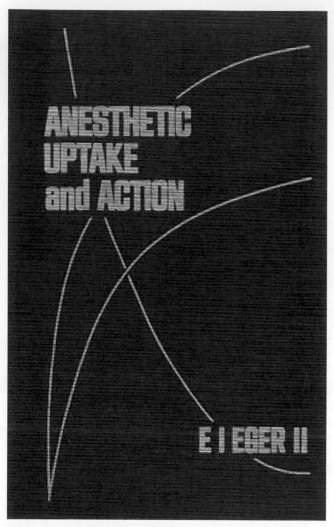

Figure 15.4   *Anesthetic Uptake and Action.*

The second book of importance, *The Pharmacology of Inhaled Anesthetics*,[4] resulted from a collaboration with James Eisenkraft and Richard Weiskopf that compiled what was known in the early 1990s of the inhaled anesthetics that were clinically important in the preceding 3 to 4 decades. It was the last of a series of books focused on inhaled anesthetics. It differed from its predecessors in having an accompanying video disc recording of 8 hours of seminars covering the material in the book with residents and student nurse anesthetists at Wake Forest University.

The recordings were produced and directed by Dirk Wales who had produced and directed less ambitious recordings of my lectures derived from earlier books. Because of my financial and professional relationship with Baxter Co., the underwriter of the book and video discs, Dirk and I were aware that these offerings would be susceptible to accusations of a bias favoring desflurane over other inhaled anesthetics, particularly sevoflurane. Accordingly, we were more than usually scrupulous in excluding such bias. We were pleased that the reviews of the offerings praised them for their objectivity:

- "Nowhere was sevoflurane denigrated, and nowhere did I think the truth was being stretched or told economically. All Baxter is getting out of this is more discussion about desflurane in the context of inhalational anesthesia in general. If that persuades anesthetists to think more about their practice and choose the best anesthetic for the clinical situation, that must be a good thing. The authors, and Dr. Eger in his seminars, have been commendably evenhanded. I have no qualms about using this material for teaching."[5]
- "…this reviewer believes that the authors have provided a balanced appraisal of the topic."[6]
- "All in all, I couldn't be much more enthusiastic about this book, particularly for the resident in training audience. It's well done. It's authoritative. And, as best I can tell, it's free."[6]

The Pharmacology of Inhaled Anesthetics continues to be used as a major resource for the education of anesthetists, particularly (as far as I can tell from interviews) of certified registered nurse anesthesia students.

My talks about this history of anesthesia led to the third book, *The Wondrous Story of Anesthesia*,[7] written over the course of 6 years. This provided another opportunity to collaborate with Larry Saidman, among my dearest friends. It also was an opportunity to collaborate with Rod Westhorpe, an Australian pediatric anesthesiologist and gifted writer and historian (**Figure 15.5**).

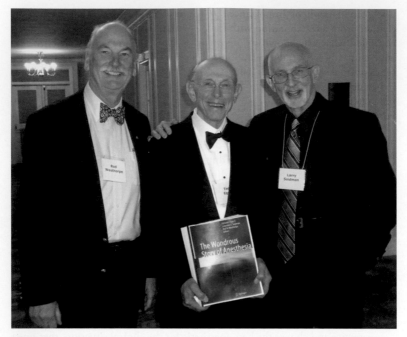

Figure 15.5   Rod Westhorpe (left), Larry Saidman (right), and me holding a copy of *Wondrous*.

The three editors wrote the first part of the book, a chronology of the evolution of anesthesia from ancient times to the present. Individual experts wrote the second part of the book, 53 chapters providing the stories of individual components of the history of anesthesia (eg, "A brief history of the patient safety movement in anesthesia").

The Wondrous Story of Anesthesia was wondrous from more than one viewpoint. It allowed the three editors to re-experience their careers. It also was timed to retrieve the stories of several others who lived the history of modern anesthesia, the period from 1950 forward, before they died.

Reflection

As I bring my autobiography to a close, I reflect on my good fortune to have been able to devote my time, energy, and affection to the two loves of my life: anesthesia and my family.

References

1. Thorwald J. *The Century of the Surgeon*. Pantheon Books, Inc; 1956.
2. Fenster JM. *Ether Day: The Strange Tale of America's Greatest Medical Discovery and the Haunted Men Who Made It*. Harper Collins; 2001.
3. Eger EI II. *Anesthetic Uptake and Action*. Williams and Wilkins; 1974.
4. Eger EI II, Eisenkraft JB, Weiskopf RB. *The Pharmacology of Inhaled Anesthetics*. Healthcare Press; 2002.
5. Lockwood GG. The pharmacology of inhaled anesthetics (A review). *Br J Anaesth*. 2003;90:261-262.
6. Egan TD. The pharmacology of inhaled anesthetics (A review). *Anesthesiology*. 2004;101:563-564.
7. Eger EI, Saidman LJ, Westhorpe R. *The Wondrous story of Anesthesia*. Springer; 2014.